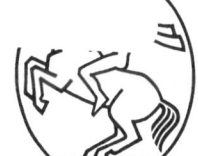

Intraoperative Doppler Sonography in Neurosurgery

Joachim M. Gilsbach

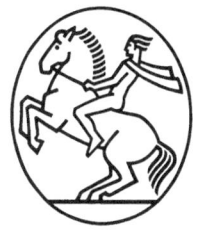

Springer-Verlag Wien GmbH

Joachim Michael Gilsbach, M. D.
Department of Neurosurgery
(Chairman: Prof. Wolfgang Seeger, M. D.)
University of Freiburg Medical School
Freiburg i. Br., Federal Republic of Germany

Supported by:
Sonderforschungsbereich Hirnforschung und
Sinnesphysiologie (SFB 70), Deutsche Forschungsgemeinschaft

With 61 Figures

Library of Congress Cataloging in Publication Data. Gilsbach, Joachim Michael. Intraoperative Doppler sonography in neurosurgery. 1. Nervous system — Surgery. 2.
Ultrasonics in surgery. I. Title. [DNLM: 1. Intraoperative complications. 2. Neurosurgery. 3. Ultrasonics — Diagnostic use. WL 368 G479i]. RD593.G46 1983.
617'.41307543. 83-20096.

ISBN 978-3-211-81768-1   ISBN 978-3-7091-4055-0 (eBook)
DOI 10.1007/978-3-7091-4055-0

Foreword

This book is written by an author whose knowledge of the subject is based on vast surgical experience.

A reliable assessment of the success or failure of a microvascular anastomosis or an aneurysm operation has until now been possible only postoperatively by angiography and transcutaneous Doppler sonography. Of particular importance are the stenoses and occlusions which can occur during the operation, but which are frequently not detected until after surgery. This induced the neurosurgeons in Freiburg, as well as those in several other hospitals, to carry out a routine control with postoperative transcutaneous Doppler following extracranial-intracranial bypass operations and angiography while still under anesthesia following aneurysm operations. The stenoses and occlusions detected were often not apparent intraoperatively. The reasons for this are that from the outside we see only the surface — and not the lumen — of a vessel, and that stenoses caused by thrombosis, indentation of the vessel wall during anastomosis or by plaque on the vessel wall are not externally obvious. Even arterial pulsation is no guarantee of patency.

The necessity to be able to detect stenoses during the operation is obvious. The microvascular Doppler sonography adopted by Dr. Gilsbach provides an expedient and safe method of recognizing such lumen narrowings. Two important innovations, the use of probes of 2 and 3 mm diameter (which is small enough to be used deep inside the subarachnoid space, particularly in the area of the Circle of Willis), and a very high frequency, make this technique ideal for very small vessels.

Doppler studies carried out by Nornes and Moritake did not meet the required degree of precision, since the size of

the probe made it impossible to exclude overlapping measurements of different vessels in deep-seated structures and
because the resolution of the equipment was not high
enough for microvessels. Gilsbach's method now enables the
surgeon to detect stenoses as a matter of routine immediately after the clipping of an aneurysm and to adjust the clip
accordingly. The same holds true for bypass operations, in
which the anastomosis can be corrected immediately in the
case of a stenosis.

In more than fifty aneurysm and thirty bypass operations
performed so far with this new control, stenoses and occlusions were detected and corrected in 10 %. Since the Doppler method is no less reliable than angiography, and has the
additional advantage of being applicable immediately after
aneurysm clipping or anastomosis (thus avoiding the
time-loss associated with wound closure and transportation
to the X-ray department for angiography) it is now preferred
in Freiburg to postoperative angiography.

The method presented enables the surgeon to make precise, repeatable, atraumatic and simple measurements of patency in the relevant vessels during the operation. In this
way he can control the surgical measures and, if necessary,
can make immediate corrections.

Freiburg im Breisgau   Prof. Wolfgang Seeger
September 1983

Acknowledgements

My grateful thanks are due to my teacher, Prof. Wolfgang Seeger, who has fostered my interest in neurosurgery and who was responsible for making these comprehensive studies possible. For their valuable assistance and constructive criticism, I am deeply indebted to my colleagues in the Department of Neurosurgery, who showed admirable patience while recordings were being made during microvascular operations, and also to Dr. Gerhard-Michael von Reutern in the Department of Clinical Neurology and Neurophysiology. I should also like to thank Mr. Hermann Kapp, who engineered the multiple modifications of the system, and Dr. D. Cathignol (INSERM, Lyon), who developed the equipment and kindly modified it to our wishes. My sincere appreciation is further due to our photographer, Gerhard Pfister, for his meticulous and numerous photographs; to our two secretaries, Vera Kullmann and Hans Foester, who suffered and forgave a great deal — particularly my handwriting; and the translators, Virginia Sonntag-O'Brien and Dr. Alec Eden. Finally, I must acknowledge the patience and understanding shown by my wife and daughter, who tolerated my mental and physical absence while this book was being prepared.

Freiburg im Breisgau   J. M. Gilsbach
September 1983

Contents

Introduction

Neurovascular surgery is a part of neurosurgery. Essentially it comprises the surgical treatment of intracranial aneurysms, the clipping of arteriovenous malformations and fistula, extracranial-intracranial revascularization surgery, and the respective animal experiments.

The goal of surgery on aneurysms and angiomas is usually to exclude them from circulation while protecting the parent and neighboring normal brain vessels. Revascularization measures are aimed at achieving better cerebral circulation by anastomozing extracranial vessels with intracranial vessels. Microsurgical skills are trained and new suture techniques are tested on laboratory animals.

The cerebral operations are performed on vessels that are often only 1 mm in size and on an organ that is extremely sensitive to ischemia. It is therefore of utmost importance that the surgical manipulation of vessels does not provoke any avoidable circulatory disturbances.

The introduction of microsurgery, through the magnified representation and improved instruments alone, has increased the safety and the precision of neurovascular operations and has considerably improved the results. Nevertheless, uncertainties and risks still exist. Under the surgical microscope it cannot be unequivocally determined as to whether a vessel was unintentionally stenosed or occluded, whether an aneurysm was incompletely clipped, and whether a microanastomosis is functioning poorly or well. The reason for these uncertainties is that the outer aspect and the inner lumen diameter do not always coincide. A number of examination methods to test intraoperatively the blood flow in the manipulated vessels were therefore tried out. However, neither the indirect methods of measuring blood flow with Xenon [34, 55, 56, 105, 106, 120], nor with thermodilution methods[32, 33], nor with fluorescein[55, 56, 105, 106], nor direct blood flow measurement using electromagnetic flow probes[39, 46, 131, 132, 173, 174, 179], anscultation[57, 58] and angiography[109, 139, 140, 142, 199], have been widely adopted for neurovascular surgery.

Ultrasound-Doppler sonography also was only rarely used intraoperatively[65, 77, 80, 124, 125, 134, 135, 136, 137], although the method has been widely adopted for transcutaneous vessel examination and although the measuring principle and the atraumatic, simple, and repeatable application of the method provides the best conditions for routine use. The reason for this was not found in the method itself but in the technical application, which was not suitable for microvascular operations.

After Freund's[64] suggestion in 1975 and after studies were carried out by Friedrich et al.[65] in 1980, which were restricted by technical limitations, the Neurosurgical Clinic of the University of Freiburg purchased a high frequency pulsed Doppler velocity meter specially developed for microvascular surgery[35, 36, 37] in order to perform systematic investigations during neurovascular operations and animal experiments.

The purpose of this book is to answer the questions as to whether ultrasound Doppler sonography can improve the results of neurovascular operations and whether this method does in fact provide the surgeon with an "intravascular eye" — even for microvessels.

Using a rat model, typical surgical findings such as local stenoses and anastomoses are controlled by Doppler sonography and angiography. Finally, the applicability and the value of the method for clinical use is discussed within the scope of two typical neurovascular operations: aneurysm and bypass surgery.

Hemodynamic Principles

The steady flow of liquids in rigid tubes is characterized by the Hagen-Poiseuille law:

$$i = \frac{\Delta p \cdot r^4 \cdot \pi}{8 \cdot \eta \cdot l} \tag{1}$$

where $i =$ the volume flow, which is measured in ml/s, $\Delta p =$ the difference between the pressure at the beginning and at the end of the tube, $r =$ the radius, $\eta =$ the viscosity, and $l =$ the length.

Of particular significance is that according to the Hagen Poiseuille law, the flow is related to the 4th power of the diameter of the tube, whereas the other factors influence it linearly.

The mean velocity of flow (v), given in cm/s, is derived from the volume flow and the radius of the vessel:

$$v = \frac{i}{\Pi \cdot r^2} \tag{2}$$

According to the law of continuity, the velocity increases as the cross-section is reduced, provided the flow volume is constant. If in the equation i is replaced with (1) the relation for the flow velocity is then:

$$v = \frac{\Delta p \cdot r^2}{8 \cdot \eta \cdot l} \tag{3}$$

These physical laws are limited in their practical biological use, particularly in the area of the brain. They only apply for a regular, laminar flow of so-called Newtonian fluids[30] in tubes with constant diameters. The arterial system, however, is made up of elastic vessels in which there is pulsatile flow and frequently changing cross-sections, pressure and resistance. Sometimes also turbulent movement of the fluid occurs. The peripheral resistance in the brain is adjusted by autoregulation in such a way that between the perfusion pressure gradients of 60 and 150 mm Hg there is constant cerebral blood flow [100, 101, 110, 203].

The velocity of the blood flow is dependent on the cardiac contractions. A flow pulse wave very similar to the pressure pulse wave arises during the cardiac cycle (Fig. 1). In contrast to the continually positive arterial pressure, however, reverse blood flow, i.e. negative flow, can occur.

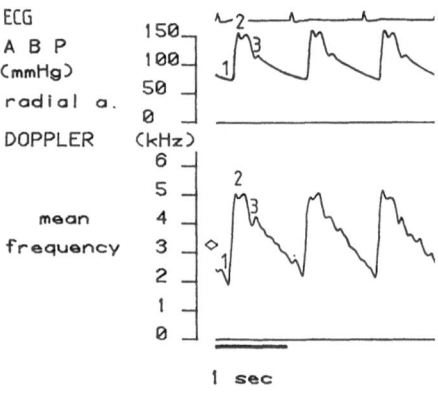

o: time averaged mean

Fig. 1. Synopsis of the pressure and flow pulse curves. *1* enddiastolic flow velocity respectively pressure, *2* systolic peak, *3* valve closure incisure

The blood flow in the arteries is essentially influenced by three basic physical properties: resistance, inertia and compliance [172]. Resistance (*R*) is caused by viscous losses of blood in the vessels. It is inversely proportional to the 4th power of the radius of the vessel and proportional to its length. To overcome this requires more than 90 % of the energy of the cardiac contractions [19].

In cerebral circulation, the pressure decreases by approximately a third as a result of resistance in vessels up to the size of the large pial arteries [9, 10, 90, 168, 183], while the remaining pressure reduction takes place in the smaller pial arteries and at the level of the arterioles.

Resistance in the cerebral blood flow is low, similar to that in the parenchymatous organs and unlike that in the muscles. Accordingly, the blood has a high diastolic flow (Figs. 30, 37, and 43).

Inertia is the impedance property mostly evident in large arteries. It represents the fact that there is a delay between the point at which the pressure increases and when the flow increases, since the mass of the blood first has to be accelerated. This hemodynamic parameter is of little significance for cerebral circulation since the arteries are relatively short.

Compliance characterizes the elasticity of the arterial wall, with which energy can be accumulated and discharged again. Compliance of the artery is responsible for the fact that peripheral perfusion takes place in diastole. This property is most pronounced in the "windkessel" function of the aorta.

Physiologically, the flow is usually laminar except in the large vessels and at the points where arteries divide. Varied flow profiles occur depending on the cross-sectional area of the artery: the flow profiles of the large vessels are relatively flat, whereas those of the smaller vessels are typically parabolic[51]. That means that in the smaller vessels, the relative number of slowly moving red blood cells increases and thus the Doppler spectrum broadens.

The stability of flow is characterized by the so-called Reynolds number (Re), a dimensionless quantity, which is approximately 2000[45].

$$Re = \frac{p \cdot D \cdot v}{\eta} \tag{4}$$

where p = density of the fluid, D = diameter of the vessel, v = flow velocity, η = absolute viscosity.

Irregular velocity distribution and pulse waves occur when there is increased acceleration or with flow impedance. After a certain velocity has been reached corresponding to a Reynolds number of approximately 2000, the flow becomes turbulent, i.e., the distribution of flow velocity becomes random.

Certain factors such as vessel curvature, caliber deviations or damage to the inner wall may cause local turbulence to occur before the velocity limit is reached[121, 177, 205].

Investigations on flow disturbances caused by stenoses have determined that there is no substantial decrease in blood flow or in poststenotic pressure until the cross-section area reduction reaches more than 80 %, a so-called critical stenosis [19, 31, 114, 116, 117, 169]. Up to this degree of narrowing, compensatory flow acceleration occurs at the site of the stenosis. Beyond the critical degree of stenosis the flow decreases at this site (Fig. 2).

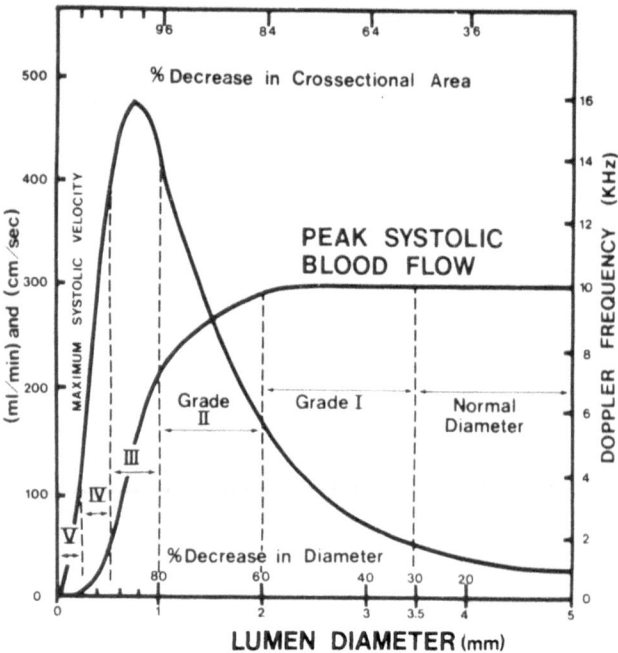

Fig. 2. Relationship between blood velocity and flow in human carotid artery stenosis, from Spencer and Reid [170]

The stenotic resistance (R)

$$R = \frac{\Delta p}{i} \tag{5}$$

where Δp = pressure difference distal and proximal to the stenosis, i = flow is dependent upon the flow, i.e., the effect of the stenosis increases as the flow increases. Conversely, a stenosis can be overlooked if, because of circulatory factors, the flow in the affected artery is unusually slow. In the case of a fixed stenosis, the narrowing must be severe before the the peripheral resistance and the blood pressure can have an effect on the stenotic resistance[163]. The resistance of these stenoses increases as the flow and the pressure increase[74, 108].

In contrast, the blood pressure and the peripheral resistance associated with dynamic stenoses are of considerable significance. When the blood pressure decreases, the cross-sectional area at the site of the stenosis is reduced and the stenotic effect is intensified. The effect of the stenosis also increases as the resistance in the periphery decreases because the velocity of flow increases at the site of the narrowing and the lateral pressure decreases. Conversely, an increase in pressure reduces the stenotic effect[99, 108, 163, 167].

Investigations into flow and mathematical models have shown that at the site of the stenosis the blood flow accelerates while the lateral pressure decreases. Distal to the stenosis there is a decrease in velocity, with turbulence and separation zones with reverse flow occurring[8, 51, 93, 200].

The behavior of flow in the human cerebral vessels, in contrast to cervical vessels, has not been thoroughly investigated. Systematic data on blood pressure, flow, and flow velocity are not available. Theoretical models for cerebral hemodynamics are also lacking[7, 68].

Ultrasound Doppler Sonography

Historical Background

The first studies on ultrasound for measurement of flow velocity in blood vessels were published 1954 by Kalmus[88] and 1957 by Baldes et al.[14]. In 1957, Satomura[164] described an ultrasound method used to inspect the function of the heart and in 1959 and 1960, he reported on its application in peripheral arteries[165, 166]. Franklin et al.[61] in 1961 published their findings of circulatory Doppler studies on animals with implanted probes. The first Doppler flowmeters used to measure blood flow velocity transcutaneously in humans were described by Baker et al.[13] in 1964 and by George et al.[70] in 1965. In 1966 Rushmer et al.[161] reported on the application of the method for examination of the carotid arteries. In the same year, Stegall et al.[176] and Strandness et al.[181] published the results of their transcutaneous studies in cases of peripheral occlusive disease.

Ultrasound Doppler sonography has become a standard medical procedure for non-invasive transcutaneous examination of blood vessels, particularly those with stenoses and occlusions in the cervical region[26, 99, 150, 172].

Technical Principle, Application, and Significance

The Doppler effect is a change in the frequency of a sound-wave when the transmitter, the receiver, or the reflecting object move towards or away from each other. The frequency change is proportional to the velocity of the movement. When the velocity of the blood flow is measured, the ultrasonic waves are emitted from a stationary transmitter, the ultrasonic probe, and are backscattered by the red blood cells which are in motion. They are received again by the probe. The frequency shift (Doppler shift) which the system perceives through the movement of the red blood cells, is expressed by the following formula:

$$F = \frac{2 \cdot Fo \cdot v \cdot \cos \alpha}{c} \tag{6}$$

where F = the Doppler frequency, Fo = the frequency of the transmitted ultrasound, v = the blood flow velocity, $\cos \alpha$ = the angle between the transmitted sound beam and the direction of the blood flow (incident angle) and c = the velocity of sound in the tissue.

The Doppler frequency is the difference between the transmitted and the received frequency and is proportional to the blood flow velocity. It is made up of a spectrum of fre-

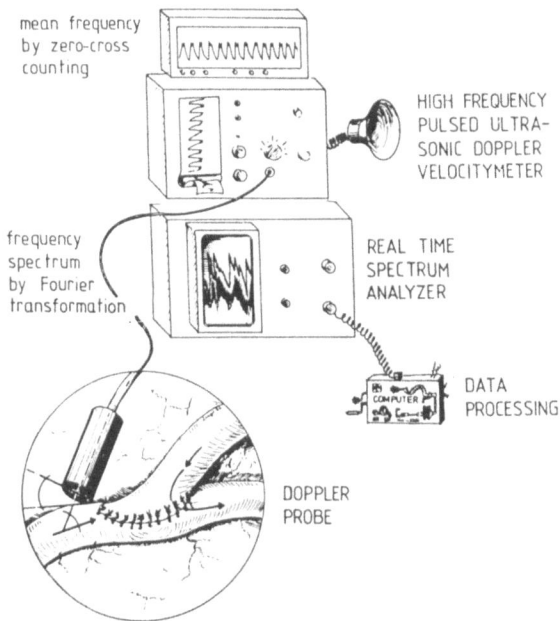

Fig. 3. Typical Doppler equipment with frequency spectrum processing systems, probe, and basic Doppler unit

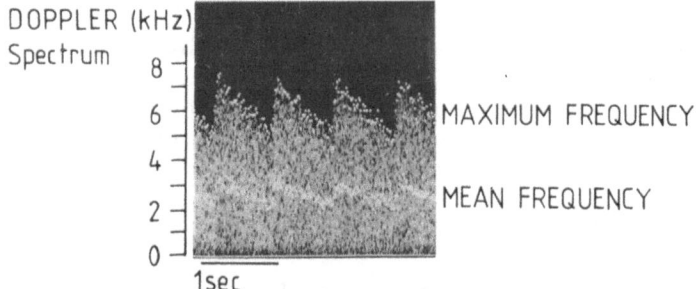

Fig. 4. Doppler frequency spectrum from a real time audiospectrum analyzer with calculated spatial mean and maximum frequencies (dotted).
The amplitude of the individual frequencies were characterized with different gray intensity

quencies (the Doppler spectrum) due to the variations in red
blood cell velocity in the flowing blood.

Turbulences, irregularities, velocity changes and flow
pulse forms can be recognized acoustically with a high degree of reliability from the Doppler freqency spectrum,
which is within the audible range[148].

The acoustic phenomenon can also be visualized, and
thus provide hard-copy documentation by means of the (audio) spectrum analysis[152], which, with the aid of electronic
circuits, makes it possible to produce a so-called real time
spectrogram. The frequencies are represented as an instan-
taneous function of time and the amplitude of each individual frequency is represented either in different shades of gray
or in various colors on a video monitor. Thus the maximum
frequency, the flow pulse waveform, and the frequency distribution can be evaluated optically (Figs. 3 and 4). Further
detailed information can be obtained by mathematical evalu-
ations of the digital data.

The reduction of the Doppler frequency spectrum to the
mean frequency by using a zero-crossing procedure has
proved easier and more economical than spectrum analysis.
The mean frequency can be registered as an analogue curve
(Fig. 5).

There is an inevitable loss of information[73], since neither
the frequency distribution, the maximum frequency, nor the

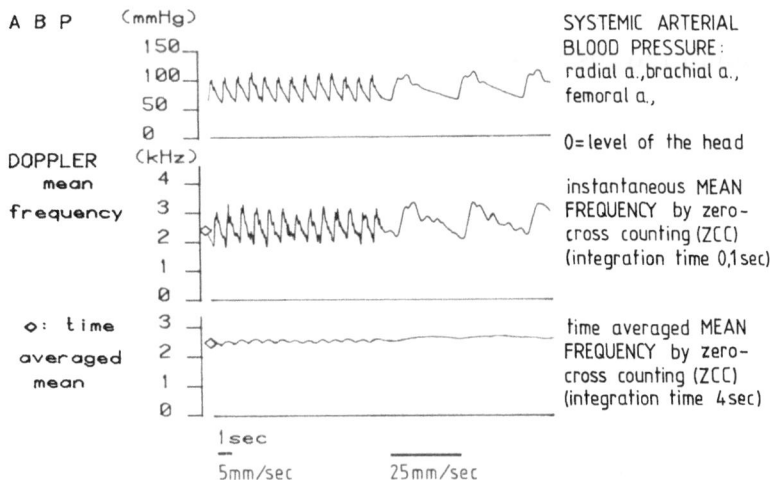

Fig. 5. Mean Doppler frequency from a zero-crosser with refernce blood pressure curves. By increasing the integration time of the analogue signal the time averaged mean frequency (temporal mean) is produced

reverse and turbulent flow can be registered. For physical reasons, this principle of measurement can incur an error of approximately 20 % in establishing the mean frequency, whereas there is only a 5 % error when the frequency change is recorded[111]. The reasons for this error include: the dependence of the zero-crossing principle on the amplitude and on the range of the Doppler frequency spectrum, the change in frequency caused by electronic processing, and changes caused by background noise[29, 111, 144, 151]. In spite of these limitations, the method has been widely accepted and yields useful, and in particular, qualitative results.

Until now, commercial Doppler sonography devices for medical use have had a transmitted frequency of between 2· and 10 MHz, depending on the medical application.

The frequency influences the depth of penetration, the power of the backscattered sound and the resolution. Absorption in the tissue is directly proportional to the frequency[182] and amounts to approx. 1 decibel damping per cm tissue thickness and per MHz transmitted frequency. Thus a recording in a depth of 1 cm when the freqency is 5 MHz shows a backscattered sound having only 1/32 of the emitted energy[148]. When the freqency is 20 MHz, less than one millionth returns to the probe.

For clinical practice this means that low frequencies are preferred for deep examinations, while for surface examinations a higher frequency is more advantageous. The higher the frequency the higher the absorption, but at the same time the better the reflection[196]. When the transmitted frequency increases, the reflected power rises, not linear but to the 4th power. Thus when the frequency rises from 5 MHz to 20 MHz, for example, the reflected power increases 256 times. Consequently, high frequencies have to be chosen for small, weakly reflecting vessels. The weak signal emitted by small transmitting crystals can also be compensated for by an increase in frequency.

The longitudinal resolution of the sound beam is affected by the electronic processing, while the lateral resolution is influenced by the frequency and the diameter of the transmitting crystal increasing as the frequency and diameter rise[76]. Therefore, if a high lateral resolution is required the transmitted frequency should be as high as possible and the crystal should have a small diameter.

The angle dependence in vitro and in vivo does not have the same influence as might be assumed from the cosinus function (Fig. 15). A Doppler effect nevertheless occurs when the incident angle is vertical, for example, and there is not a maximum effect when the incident angle is orthograde. This is due partially to the divergence of the sound of the transmitting crystal and partially to the various directions in which the red blood cells reflect the sound. Experimental studies carried out by Kaneko et al.[89] using a 5 MHz ultrasound device show, for example, neither an essential change in flow velocity nor an alteration in flow patterns when the angle between the sound axis and the flow direction is between 30 and 70 degrees.

The velocity of sound in the blood is dependent upon the temperature, the amount of protein, and the hematocrit value. However, whith normal temperatures and a hematocrit of 30—50 %, these differences can be ignored, allowing one to assume a constant velocity of approximately 1550 m/s[22].

In most Doppler instruments used for routine diagnosis, one crystal usually transmits the ultrasonic beam and another continuously receives the backscattered sound. These are called CW (continuous wave) Doppler instruments. Using this technique, every movement in the area taken in by the wide and deep-reaching sound beam is registered. Because inaccuracies can result from the overlapping of arteries, it is not possible to examine one individual vessel in isolation by fading out the surroundings. All of the different velocities occurring in the cross-sectional area of the examined vessel are registered.

To solve this problem, a pulsed Doppler system can be used, in which the ultrasound is alternately transmitted and received, mostly via one single crystal. So-called electronic gate systems enable the investigation of a selective sample volume, which can be varied in its size as well as in its distance from the probe [11, 12, 144]. The sample volumina are usually club shaped, with the handle of the club pointing towards the probe. When the electronic gate is moved through a vessel, flow profiles can be produced (Fig. 6).

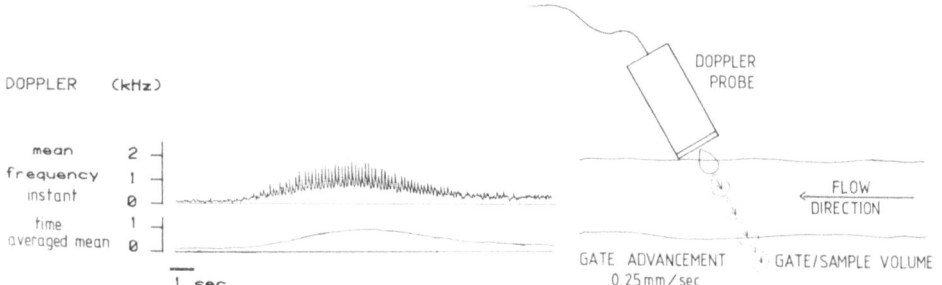

Fig. 6. Flow profile generated by continuous advancement of an electronic gate through the vessel. If the angle, the site, and the velocity of the gate are known, it is possible to estimate the diameter

Using a multi-gate system, in which simultaneously functioning electronic gates are positioned next to each other, it is possible to detect flow profile changes across the vessel diameter during the cardiac cycle [4, 5, 24, 81, 92, 113].

With a single gate having the same diameter as the vessel, the average velocity taken from the entire cross-sectional area of the vessel can be determined. With smaller gates, only the average velocity in the sample volume (spatial mean), i.e., at one site within the vessel, can be recorded (Fig. 7).

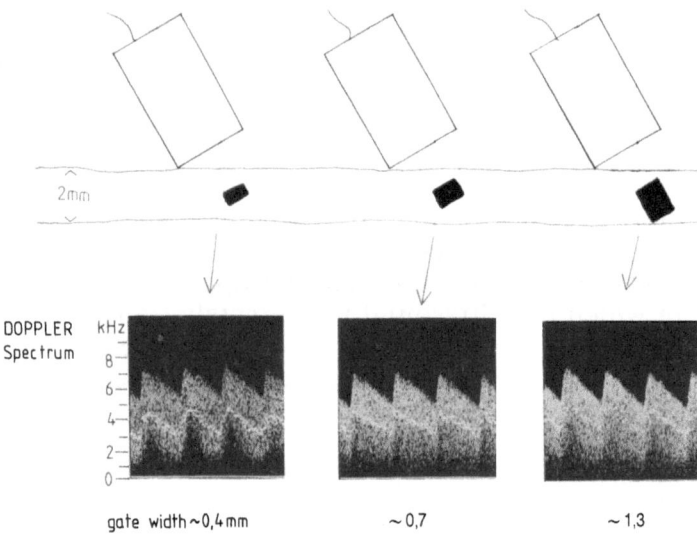

Fig. 7. The 3 primarily used gates of the microvascular Doppler system. Note the relatively uniform spectrum of the 3 different sized sample volumina. This is due to the flat profile of the investigated angioma vessel and the relatively large lateral diameter of the gates. The mean frequencies in the sample volumina i. e. the spatial mean frequencies, are space averaged, whereas mean frequencies in one or more cardiac cycle, i. e. the temporal mean, are time averaged

When the gates are very small in relation to the vessel, the inner diameter of the artery can be determined approximately by continuous gate shifting, provided the angle is known[75] (Fig. 6).

The pulse repetition frequency characterizes the time intervals between the individual sound pulses. It puts a limit on the Doppler frequency that can be detected and determines, along with the sound absorption, how deep the recordings can be made. The higher the repetition frequency, the lower the measuring depth and the higher the maximum detectable Doppler frequency (at most, half the repetition frequency). For example, when the repetition frequency is 25 kHz, the maximum Doppler frequency that can be obtained without so called "aliasing" is 12.5 kHz[150].

The direction of the blood can be determined electronically according to whether the received frequency is higher or lower than the emitted frequency[112].

An essential component of the probe is the transmitting crystal. These crystals are not monocrystals but usually polycrystal ceramics, e.g., lead zirconium titanate[148, 195]. The sound energy emitted is directly proportional to the surface area of the crystal and is proportional to the transmitted frequency to the fourth power.

The probe is used transcutaneously or is placed intraoperatively directly on the vessel at a 40—60 degree angle to the direction of flow. This angle effects the optimum intensity and frequency of the Doppler signal. In cases of freely dissected vessels, the probe can be secured with cuffs at a defined angle to the flow direction in order to avoid inaccuracy due to angle variation[195]. However, the advantage of Doppler sonography, namely the ability to make atraumatic recordings over an entire vessel, is then sacrificed in favor of precision of measurement.

Apart from providing information on the presence and the direction of blood flow, the Doppler method also establishes the velocity of the red blood cells in their spatial and temporal distribution. Information can thus be obtained not only on the average velocity, but also on the distribution of the velocity within the vessel. It is possible to separate the laminar flow from an irregular and turbulent flow and thus to detect localized or systemic disturbances of the blood movement by acceleration or wall irregularities.

The velocity changes within the cardiac cycle, the so-called flow pulse waves, also indicate by their form local and systemic changes of resistance. Clinically, the resistance index introduced by Pourcelot[147] has proved useful for estimating the peripheral flow resistance; e.g., a relative reduction of the pulsatile amplitude indicates a decrease in resistance (Figs. 8, 30, 37, 42 and 43).

Recordings made at various sites with the angle kept as constant as possible enable separation of local and systemic changes by comparing the flow pulse waves and the Doppler spectra. Furthermore, narrowings can be established and quantified on the basis of local acceleration.

The major importance of transcutaneous Doppler sonography in neurology and neurosurgery is the diagnosis of arterial disease in the area of the cervical vessels[26, 172]. The method can also provide information on intracranial pathological changes, e.g. in cases of angiomas[50, 154], of traumatic intracra-

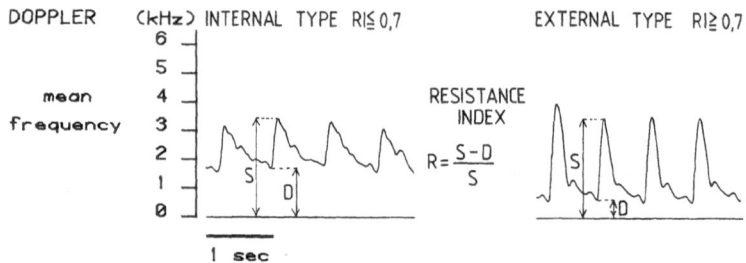

Fig. 8. Resistance index as a sign of the relative size of the amplitude of the flow pulse curve. Left: typical low resistance in intracerebral circulation, right: high resistance in peripheral circulation

nial pressure increase[178], of changes in intracranial resistance by hypo- or hyperventilation[16], and of intracranial circulatory arrest[27, 59, 104, 133]. Occlusion of the sinus cavernous fistula with a balloon catheter can also be controlled by Doppler sonography[28, 115].

Within the scope of extracranial — intracranial bypass surgery, numerous studies have been reported on the aid of Doppler sonography in determining the position of the donor artery and in examining the patency and the flow after surgery (see chapter on Bypass).

During neurosurgical procedures in which the patient is kept in a sitting position, the precordial ultrasound Doppler recording is an indispensible method for the early detection of air-embolism[38, 72].

Direct recordings carried out intraoperatively have been described for carotid endarterectomies[119, 175], for extracranial — intracranial bypass operations (see chapter on Bypass), for clipping of aneurysms of the circle of Willis (see chapter on Aneurysms), for operations on angiomas[80, 136, 137], for patency testing of the superior longitudinal sinus[25], and for the testing of microvascular experimental anastomoses (see chapter on Anastomoses).

Doppler Device

Introduction

The neurosurgical application of the intraoperative Doppler examination method requires a Doppler system which can record manipulated vessels of less than 1 millimeter in diameter. The system must also enable examinations to be carried out under visual control, with direct contact between the probe and the vessel and in the narrow space at the base of the brain. It must be able to record discretely vessels which are closely adjacent.

Only a pulsed technique with a high transmitted frequency meets these requirements. Neither the 4 MHz nor the 5 MHz CW commercial Doppler instruments used by Brawley[25], Friedrich et al.[65] and Moritake et al.[124] fulfills the con-

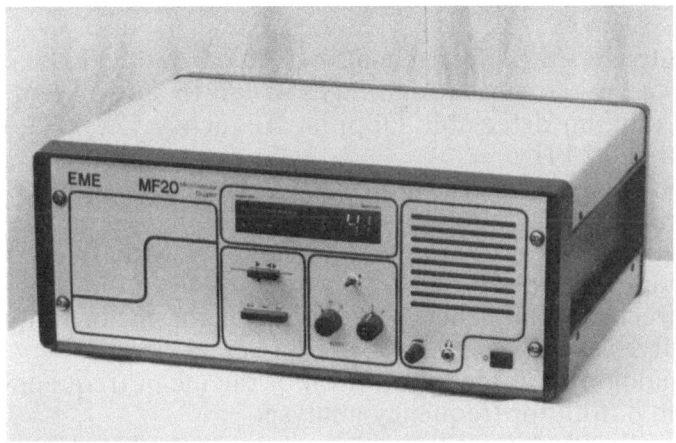

Fig. 9. The present appearance of the microvascular Doppler system MF 20 (original name of the prototype: Microflo) Eden Medizinische Elektronik GmbH, D-7770 Überlingen

ditions listed above. Nornes et al. [134, 135] used a pulsed Doppler instrument having a transmitted frequency of 6 and 10 MHz and relatively small probes. However, since only results were published of examinations performed on large intracranial arterial main stems and angioma arteries, and none on vessels smaller than 1 mm in diameter, this device also has its limitations.

For our studies we selected a prototype of a pulsed Doppler ultrasound instrument with a transmission frequency of 20 MHz developed by Cathignol [35, 36] (Fig. 9). It was similar to a system used in the United States for experimental and clinical studies [20, 21, 54, 62, 63, 78].

Technical Data

- pulsed ultrasonic Doppler velocity meter (MF 20) (Figs. 9 and 10)
- transmitted frequency 20 MHz
- pulse durations of 250, 450, 850, 1500 ns corresponding to axial gate width of approximately 0.4, 0.7, 1.3, and 2.3 mm (axial resolution)
- lateral gate width (lateral resolution): 1.1 mm with the 3 mm probe
- automatic gate shifting in 0.1 mm steps with a velocity of 0.25 mm/s
- pulse repetiton frequencies of 100, 50 and 25 kHz, corresponding to measuring ranges of 7.5, 15, and 30 mm
- maximum detectable Doppler frequency 12.5 kHz, minimum 0.1 kHz
- mean frequency by built-in zero-crosser, integration time 0.1—4.0 s
- calibration by a frequency generator with fixed 1 kHz Doppler freqency
- direction established by reversal of the mean frequency curves
- analog output for registration of the mean frequency, audio output for frequency analysis
- sterilizable miniature probes, 1 cm long, 2 and 3 mm diameter (Fig. 11)
- frequency spectrum analysis in real time with FFT (Angioscan) (Fig. 10)

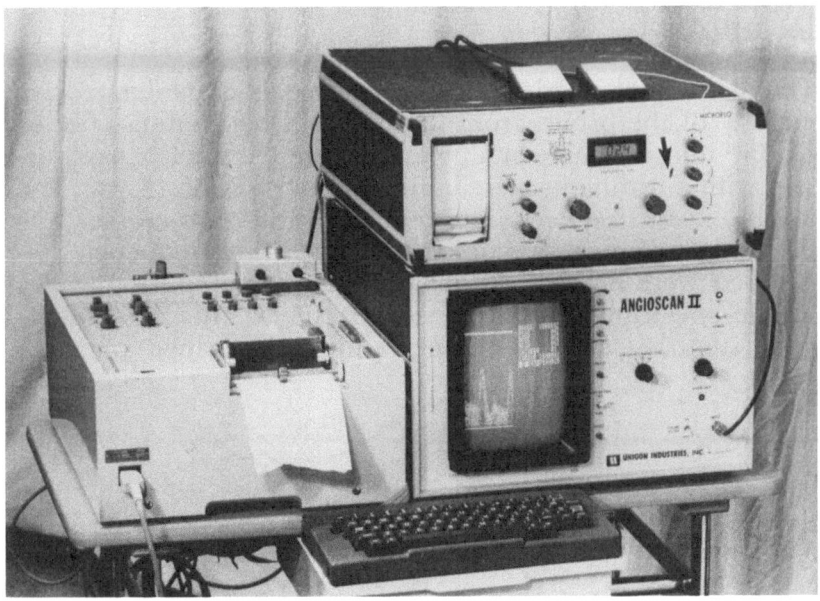

Fig. 10. Doppler equipment: high frequency pulsed Doppler velocity meter (Microflo), real time frequency analyzer (Angioscan II), and ink recorder (Cardirex 4 T) for mean frequency curve registration

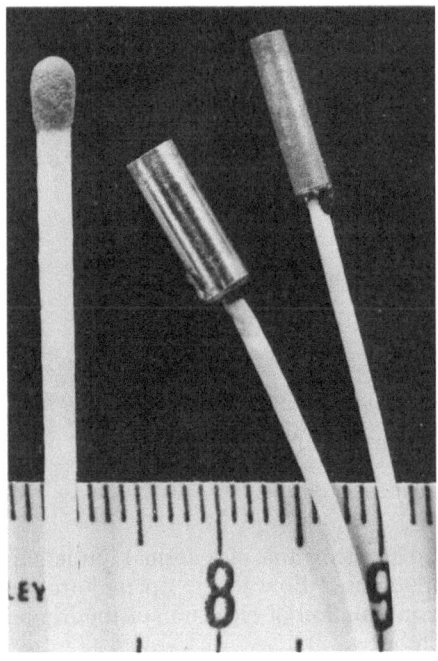

Fig. 11. Doppler probes: external diameter 3 or 2 mm, probe length 1 cm

Results

The instrument is able to record all vessels in the immediate vicinity of the probe, from the pial and perforating arteries of 0.15 mm in diameter upwards to the cervical carotid artery with a width of several millimeters (Figs. 12, 13, 44). The lowest mean frequency registered with the zero-crosser was 0.2 kHz. In clinical practice the highest mean frequencies registered were 8 kHz. The maximum detectable frequencies in the spectrum seldom exceeded 10 kHz. In cases of severe stenoses and av-malformations, the range of mea-

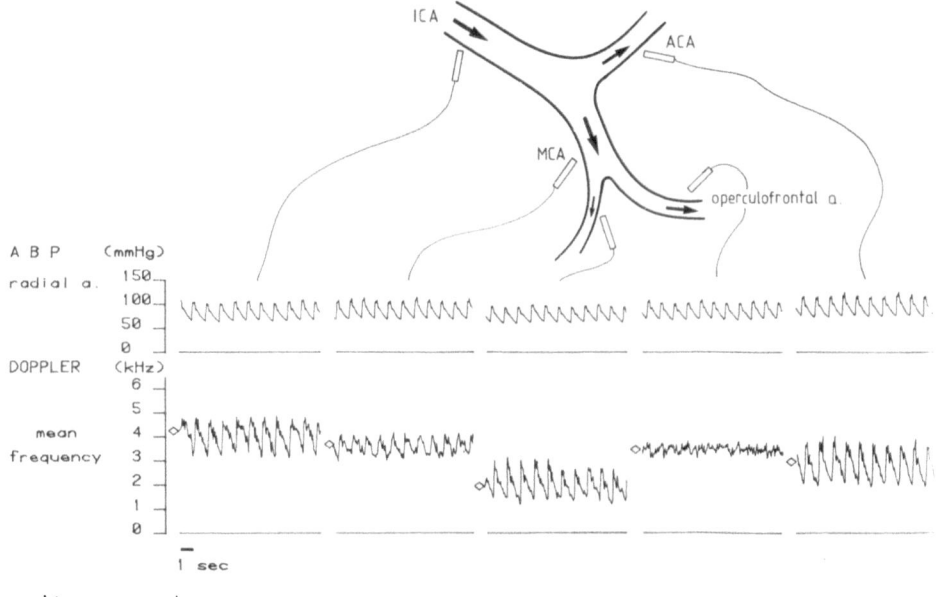

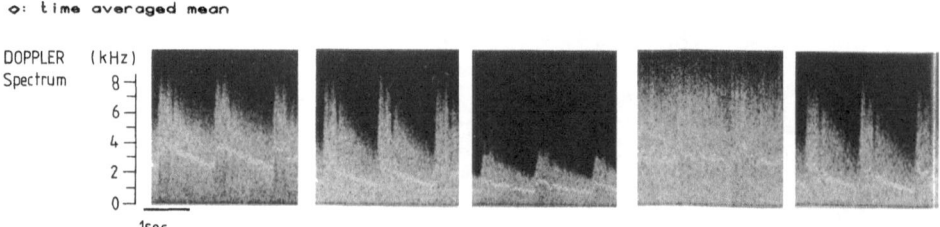

Fig. 12. Mean frequency curves and spectrograms of a normal intracranial vessel tree. Note the high, unmodulated flow in the operculofrontal branch due to hyperemia after discontinuation of retraction of the frontal lobe

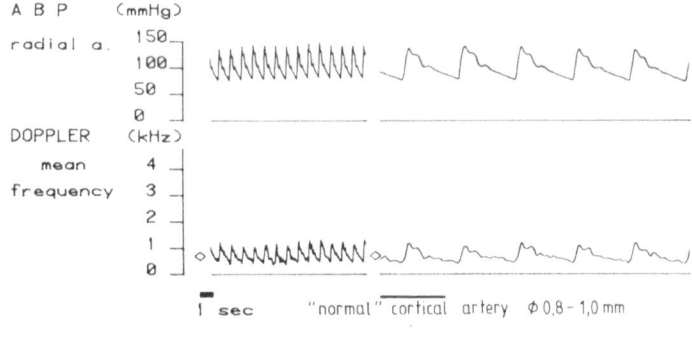

Fig. 13. Normal flow pattern of a small cortical artery

surement was exceeded, which could be recognized from the truncated systolic curves.

The vessels were examined using mainly 0.4 or 0.7 mm gates, since these produced the fewest disturbances and provide the most precise flow patterns. This resulted in the Doppler frequencies among the smaller vessels being proportional to the mean velocity in the entire vessel. Vessels of approximately 1.5 mm in diameter and larger showed a preference for higher frequencies in the spectrum, while relatively homogeneous frequencies occured in smaller vessels. Accordingly, the flow profiles of the smaller vessels were more pointed, whereas those of the larger vessels were flatter.

Discussion

Our studies support the findings of Blair et al.[20, 21], Freed et al.[62, 63], Greene et al.[75], and Hartely and Cole[78], which establish a transmitted frequency of 20 MHz as prerequisite for recording microvessels. The disadvantage of high transmitted frequency, namely, the limited penetration depth, affects only transcutaneous examinations and limits the penetration depth to approximately 1.5 cm.

It is difficult to obtain a valid velocity profile using the pulsed technique of our system because the gates are relatively large in relation to the cross-sections of the microvessels, which can produce inaccuracies[87]. The same applies for determining the inner diameter of the vessel from the profiles[20, 21, 54]. Angle error is an additional source of inaccuracy.

These restrictions do not pertain to most clinical questions regarding the patency, the direction and velocity distribution or changes of flow. Nevertheless, more accurate spectrum analyses are required for future applications, facilitating comparative studies, information storage and quantitative assessment.

Conclusions

Using the high frequency pulsed Doppler system in the field of neurosurgery, vessels ranging in size from the perforating arteries up to the common carotid artery can be examined intraoperatively. In these vessels the mean Doppler frequencies are usually between 0.2 and 10 kHz. Patency, direction of flow, laminar and non-laminar flow and alterations in flow velocity are detectable from the mean frequency curve from the zero-crosser. The profiles and measurements obtained from the cross-section of the vessel are not precise, since the measurement ranges are relatively large in relation to the vessel.

Laboratory Animal Model

Introduction

There are no extensive reports on the typical intraoperative Doppler findings of microvessels in the presence of local or systemic hemodynamic changes, caused, for example, by stenoses or hyperemia, under standardized conditions. Only one report[63] deals with the detection and grading of microvascular stenoses. Nevertheless there is a need to establish characteristic microvascular Doppler findings, both in normal and impaired flow conditions, in order to evaluate the quality of microsurgical procedures. The findings in large vessels cannot be transferred to small arteries without further investigations.

The carotid artery of the rat serves well as a model for obtaining controlled data: it has a diameter of 1 mm, which is the size most commonly found in microvascular surgery, its flow velocity is comparable to that of brain vessels of the same size, and there is adequate information available for carrying out dissection and anastomoses.

In order to familiarize oneself with the methodology, one should determine Doppler sonographic normal findings and typical changes caused by variations in pressure and resistance in order to be able to distinguish them later from local changes brought on surgically. Since in practice stenoses often cause considerable problems, it is important to know at what degree of lumen narrowing the stenosis can be recognized by Doppler sonography and also whether and at what stage characteristic pulse waveforms and velocity changes appear as the vascular system is impeded.

Material and Method

The findings are based on recordings made on rats weighing 250—400 g. The animals, which breathed spontaneously, were anesthetized intraperitoneally with pentobarbital sodium (40 mg/kg body weight) or (0.5—1.5 ml) Thalamonal and were heparinized. The arterial blood pressure was measured either via the cannulated external carotid artery, the brachial artery or the axillary artery, or via the femoral artery or abdominal aorta, all of which were also used as angiographical approaches.

Animal Models

Three models have proved useful and effective for the various investigations (Fig. 14):

1. The right common carotid artery for stenoses and end-to-end anastomoses. It can be well visualized by retrograde angiography via the brachial artery and pressure can be measured proximal and distal to the stenosis while the external carotid artery is additionally cannulated.

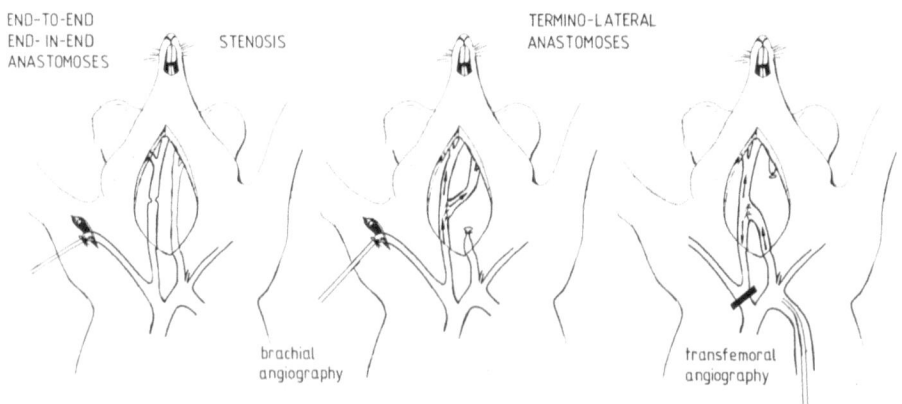

Fig. 14. Microsurgical measures performed on the carotid artery of the rat, which are suitable for angiographically controlled Doppler sonographic examinations

2. The y-shaped connection of the left with the right common carotid artery for end-to-side anastomosis[158, 159]. It too, is demonstrated angiographically via the brachial artery.

3. The h-shaped connection with proximal ligation of the brachiocephalic trunk, which is demonstrated via the aorta[42, 179].

Normal Findings

The flow pulse waveforms in the common carotid artery of the rat closely follow the pressure pulse waveforms (Figs. 16 and 17). The diastolic flow is relatively low, the resistance index is 0.76—0.95. The time averaged mean Doppler frequencies are between 0.8 to 1.3 kHz when the inner diameters (angiographically ascertained) are 0.9 to 1.2 mm and the mean arterial blood pressure levels range from 50 to 130 mm Hg. The maximum systolic mean Doppler frequency is about 2.7 kHz where the minimal mean diastolic frequencies are about 0.1 kHz. Mechanical irritations during dissection as well as exsiccation cause the mean flow velocity to increase and the pulse amplitude to decrease.

Angle Dependence

The angle between the beam of ultrasound and the direction of flow of between 40 and 60 degrees (average 50 degrees) provides the best recording conditions, yields the highest mean frequencies from the zero-crosser and the slightest frequency differences (Fig. 15).

Resistance Change

An increase in the peripheral or the cerebral resistance can be recognized from a decrease in the diastolic flow velocity to approximately 0 and from steep, small-peaked pulse waveforms (Fig. 16). When there is a reduction of the peripheral resistance after vasodilatation, e.g., with sodium nitroprusside, an increase in the amplitude modulation and

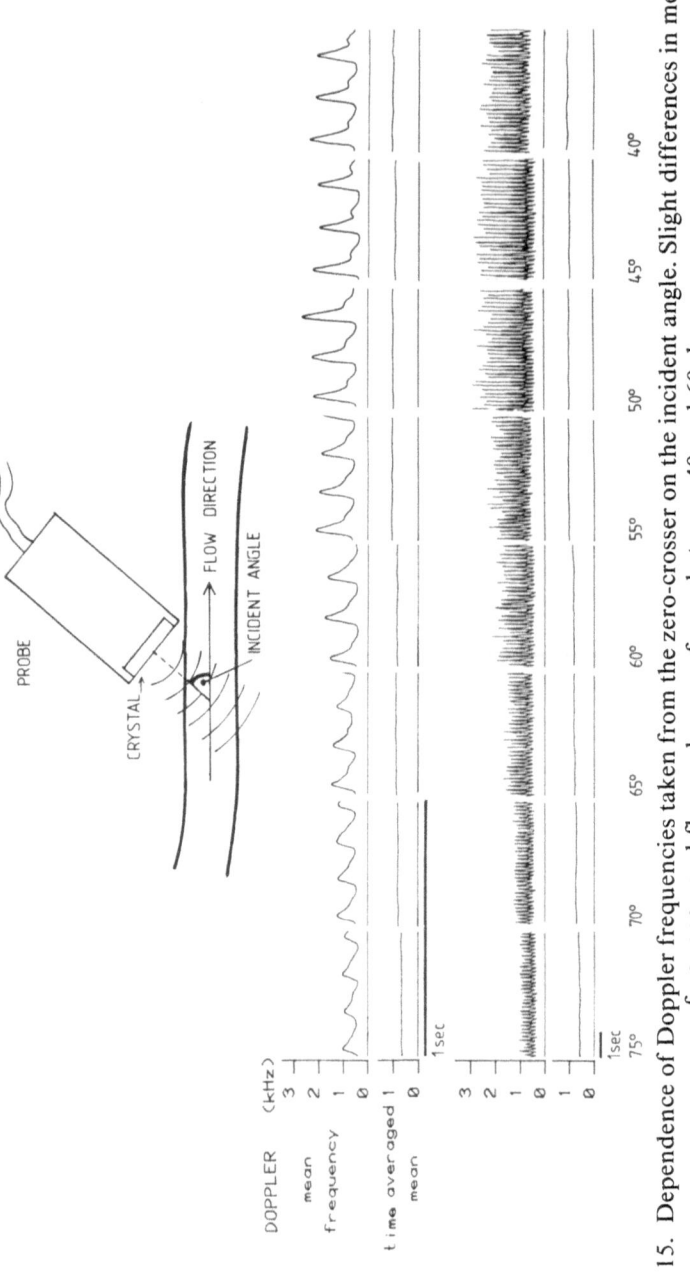

Fig. 15. Dependence of Doppler frequencies taken from the zero-crosser on the incident angle. Slight differences in mean frequency and flow pulse waveforms between 40 and 60 degrees

in the mean flow velocity can occur when a drop in pressure takes place. After sodium nitroprusside administration has been terminated and there is reactive hypertension and continued low resistance, the pulse waveforms become irregular with a slight amplitude modulation and a high diastolic flow (Fig. 17).

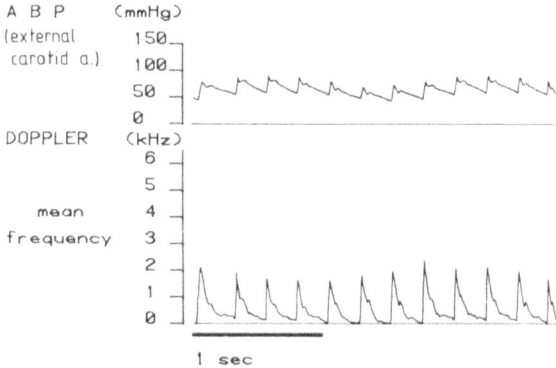

Fig. 16. Flow pulse waves in the common carotid artery of the rat during peripheral (cerebral) resistance increase with a steep systolic peak and little diastolic flow

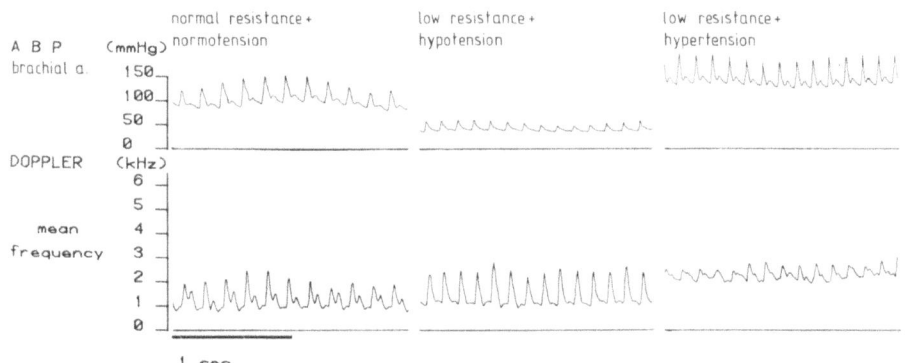

Fig. 17. Left: flow patterns in normal pressure and resistance; middle: flow patterns in low pressure and low resistance following injection of sodium nitroprusside. Right: flow pattern in the phase of hypertensive reaction after discontinuing the drug induced hypotension with persisting low resistance and therefore hyperperfusion

Stenoses

Standardized circular stenoses with a 10×10 thread which extend over a short distance allow a comparison to be made of the Doppler sonographic degree of stenosis $= 100 \times$ (1-Doppler frequency proximal to the stenosis : Doppler frequency at the stenosis) with the angiographic degree of the stenosis $= 100 \times$ (1-cross sectional area of the stenosis : cross sectional area proximal to the stenosis). Flow acceleration can be registered by Doppler sonography if there is a lumen area reduction of roughly 40 % or more. Here a Doppler underestimation of the narrowing has to be reckoned with. However, the degree of inaccuracy decreases from about 30 % to 15 % as the degree of stenosis increases.

The results with this type of stenosis have shown that when the Doppler grading of a stenosis is less than 30 %, angiography registers narrowing of 38—52 %; a 30—60 % lumen area reduction estimated by Doppler corresponds to 49—78 % in angiography, and 60—80 % in Doppler corresponds to 60—90 % in angiography.

For microvessels, the time averaged mean frequency proved to be the most precise and most reliable parameter for stenosis grading, followed by the systolic mean frequency.

Stenoses can also be recognized from typical changes in the pulse waveforms. Slight lumen reductions of 30—60 % show a rise of the systolic and diastolic level at the site of the stenosis while the pulse waves remain undisturbed proximal and distal to the stenosis. Narrowings of between 60 and 80 % show distinctly broadened and raised curves during systole or double-peaked pulse waveforms at the site of the stenosis. Flow accelerations a few millimeters distal to the site of the stenosis can still be observed. Severe stenoses of over 80 % show a pulse amplitude which is markedly lower proximal to the stenosis — and even more pronounced behind it — in comparison with normal findings. Flow velocity on the whole is reduced. At the site of the stenosis itself, when the velocity is still high, a round, mostly irregular pulse waveform can be recorded. As the narrowing increases and the flow decreases, this pulse waveform changes into a barely modulated pulse wave with slight acceleration (Figs. 18 and 19).

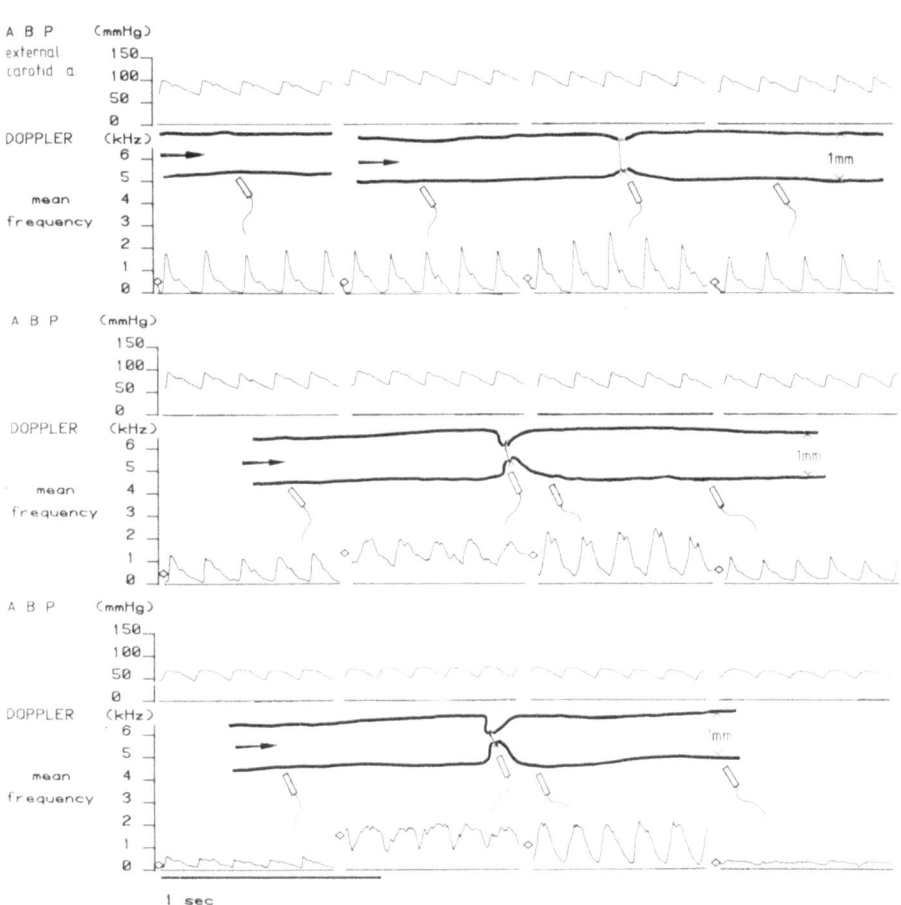

o: time averaged mean

Fig. 18

Figs. 18 and 19. Mean frequency curves and spectra for various degrees of short stenoses made with a thread. Top: slight narrowing, less than 60 % reduction of cross-sectional area; middle: moderate, 60—80 % stenosis; bottom: severe stenosis, more than 80 %

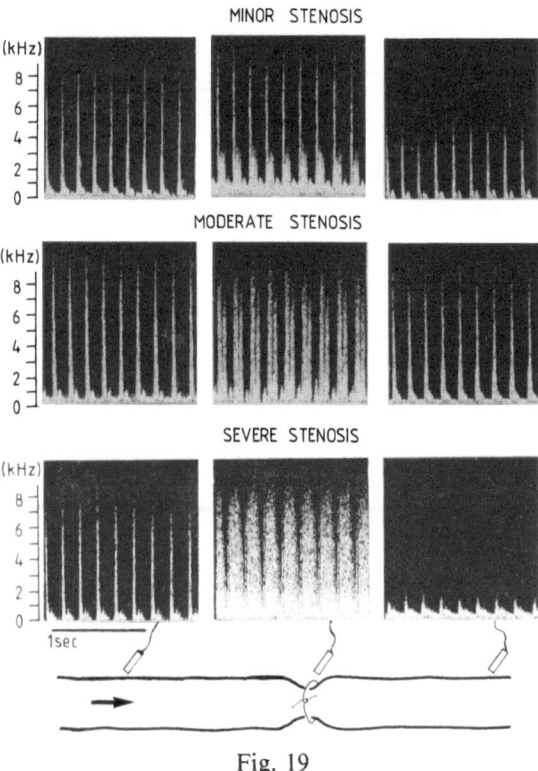

Fig. 19

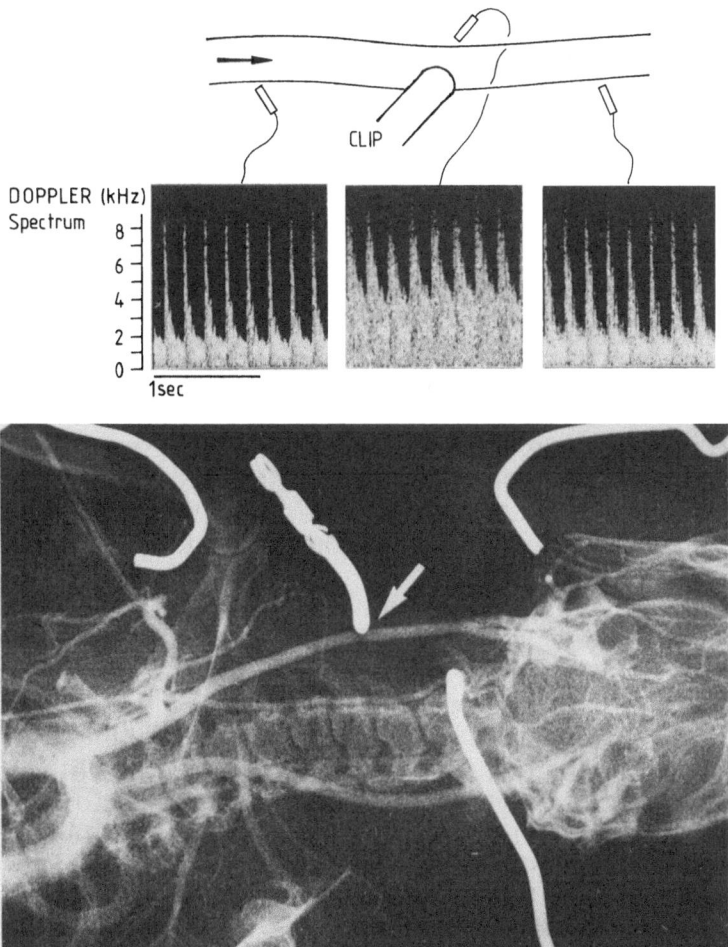

Fig. 20. Doppler spectra for lateral stenosis of the common carotid artery
of a rat with an aneurysm clip. Findings indicate slight to moderate stenosis

The example of a marginal narrowing by an aneurysmal
clip shows that in this surgery-like case the hemodynamic effect of a stenosis can be detected and quantified (Fig. 20).

Discussion

Resistance and pressure changes in microvessels can be registered just as in large vessels. The angle dependency of the Doppler shift is minimal when the vessels can be seen and the probe angle is adjusted under optic and/or acoustic control. This has been substantiated by studies carried out by Eldridge et al. [54] using a similar device. The conversion of the frequency shift into velocities, which is often practiced [20, 21, 54], yields no additional information and is not precise because there is no other reliable method for obtaining a practicable velocity calibration necessary for quantification in the investigated vessels.

It is therefore recommended that comparative studies and an evaluation of the pulse waveforms should be carried out, in which the error associated with angle variation and the lack of precision in measuring the frequencies do not play an essential role.

Thread stenoses are not equivalent to naturally occurring stenoses. However, they can be easily controlled on one plane by angiography and represent the shortest possible narrowing, and thus the most difficult to detect.

In the area of the stenosis, the axial and lateral extension of the measuring range makes Doppler recording of the narrowest point in isolation impossible. Accordingly, overlappings occur in regions of slower or retrograde flow and result in an underestimation of the stenosis. Another possible error is a reduction of flow by shock, for instance, which leads to accelerations typical for a less severe stenosis.

Conclusions

It is possible to carry out Doppler sonographic investigations on the common carotid artery of the rat, which has a diameter of approximately 1 mm. Hemodynamically effective alterations in resistance and pressure can be recognized from the typical flow pattern changes. Circular stenoses of small length can be detected by Doppler sonography from a cross-section reduction of about 40 % upward and can be graded according to velocity increase and pulse waveform.

Experimental Microvascular Anastomoses

Introduction

The quality of microvascular anastomoses is usually evaluated according to the following criteria: patency rate , which is more than 90 %[2, 189], morphological examinations[43, 97], blood flow measurements[128], and the inspection of the outer aspect or mechanical patency tests[1, 79].

Electromagnetic flow measurements are not often reported[15, 179, 194] and angiography is seldom used, either immediately following the anastomosis or after a period of some days[40, 42, 157, 189, 190, 198].

Direct Doppler sonographic examinations of microvascular anastomoses have not been widely used up till now because of the lack of commercially available equipment suitable for use on tiny vessels[17, 44]. Studies do exist, however, on a 20 MHz system with high resolution[78], with which flow in microvessels can be recorded without any problem[21, 63].

With our method it is possible to record not only the patency and the flow velocity in all the branches, but also the local hemodynamics in the area of anastomosis. This enables intraoperative evaluation of the quality of an anastomosis and the various anastomotic techniques.

Material and Method

The findings are based on 15 end-to-end, 15 end-in-end, and 15 end-to-side anastomoses performed on the carotid artery of rats. They were carried out with single knot sutures without the use of fibrin glue. Approximately 20 minutes after circulation was re-established, the anastomoses were examined and controlled angiographically.

Examination Procedure

The following routine examination procedure following microvascular anastomoses is recommended (Table 1):

Table 1. *Routine procedure steps for microvascular experimental anastomoses*

vessel section studied	information/reason for study
proximal branch site of clip	local acceleration caused by swelling due to temporary clip
proximal branch	patency, flow direction and flow velocity, pulse waveform
anastomosis center	acceleration, irregularities and turbulences due to narrowing and vessel wall irregularities
transition region between donor and recipient artery	acceleration, irregularities and turbulences as result of type of anastomosis, narrowing, and vessel wall irregularities
distal branch near the anastomosis	acceleration extending beyond the area of the anastomosis
distal branch (branches)	patency, flow direction, flow velocity, pulse waveform, comparison with proximal branch
distal branch (branches) site of clip	local acceleration caused by swelling due to temporary clip

The best recording conditions are archieved with a probe-vessel angle of approximately 50 degrees with direct probe contact, acoustic coupling by means of a drop of a sodium chloride solution or blood, and 0.7—1.3 mm gate. For a rat heart rate of 300 beats per minute, paper velocity should be adjusted for analog registration of the mean frequency curves of 10 and 100 mm/s.

End-to-end Anastomoses

As a rule, end-to-end anastomoses with approximately 8 sutures in a vessel with an inner diameter of 0.9—1.0 mm are

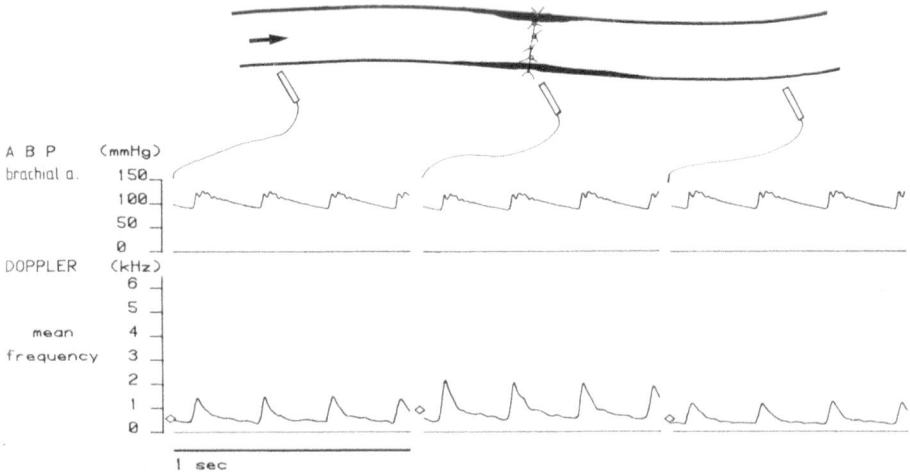

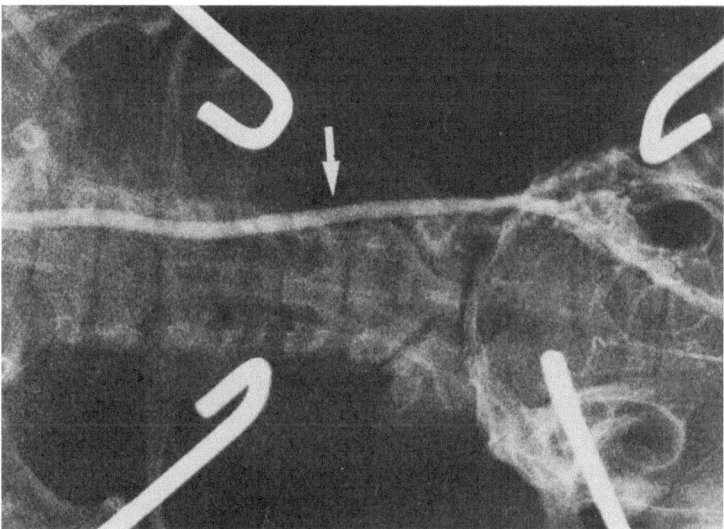

Fig. 21. End-to-end anastomosis on the common carotid artery of the rat. Doppler sonography shows only slight acceleration at the site of the anastomosis. Normal flow patterns as sign of hemodynamically satisfactory anastomosis. (Arrow: region of the anastomosis)

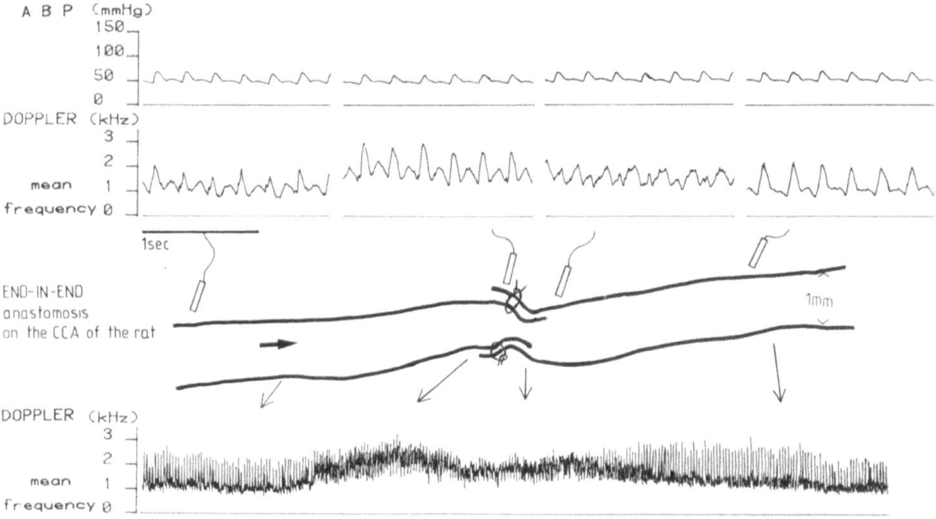

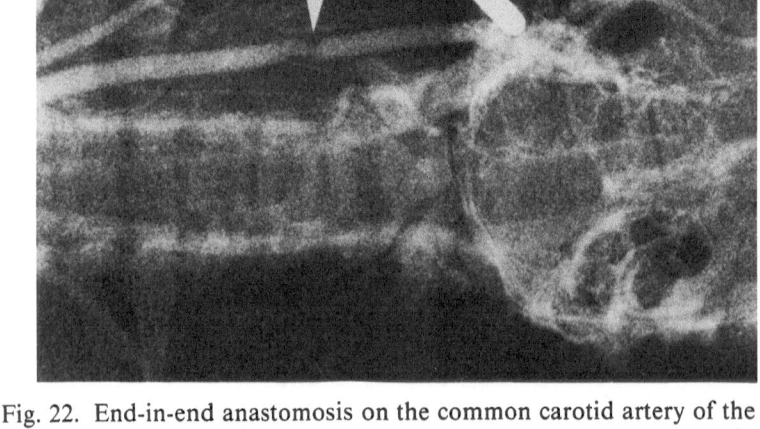

Fig. 22. End-in-end anastomosis on the common carotid artery of the rat. Doppler sonography shows flow irregularities and marked acceleration as a sign of hemodynamically unsatisfactory anastomosis. The flow pattern along the bottom of the diagram results from continuous displacement of the probe along the longitudinal axis of the vessel. (Arrow: region of the anastomosis)

open, provided the microvascular surgeon possesses sufficient technical skill. In the area of the anastomosis, however,
flow acceleration can be established which corresponds to
an angiographically detectable stenosis. The degree of stenosis which is determined from the acceleration is usually between 20 and 40 % when the anastomosis is properly functioning. Flow pulse curves with systolic and diastolic increase in amplitude modulation are characteristic (Figs. 21
and 27).

In the case of severe stenosis, m-shaped curve patterns
and irregular flow pulse waveforms occur, which can also be
established a few millimeters distal to the anastomosis (Figs.
22 and 23). Rapid flow velocity can result from swelling of
the intimal and medial wall layers at the site of the temporary clip and is easily mistaken for a good flow, since the caliber of the vessel shows no outward change (Fig. 25).

End-in-end Anastomoses

The degree of local stenosis during end-in-end anastomosis
varies according to the technique used. Anastomotic occlusions and severe stenoses are generally more often associated with end-in-end anastomoses than with end-to-end anastomoses. The average degree of stenosis of patent anastomoses ranges from 20 to 60 % (Figs. 22, 23 and 27).

End-to-side Anastomoses

In the model with right sided main stem (Figs. 24 and 25),
the flow division shows a preference for the left side.

The anastomoses with an oblique incision of the lateral
branch and with 8 to 10 knots show marked acceleration in
the areas proximal or distal to the anastomoses as a result of
stenoses (Fig. 24). In contrast, the anastomoses carried out
according to the patch technique inconstantly demonstrate
acceleration in the acute angle area of the bifurcation (Fig.
25).

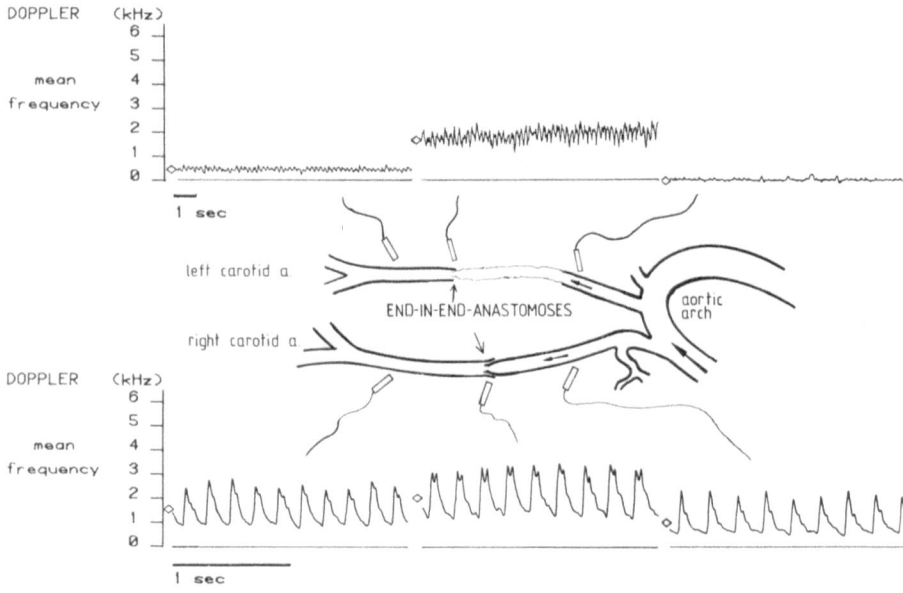

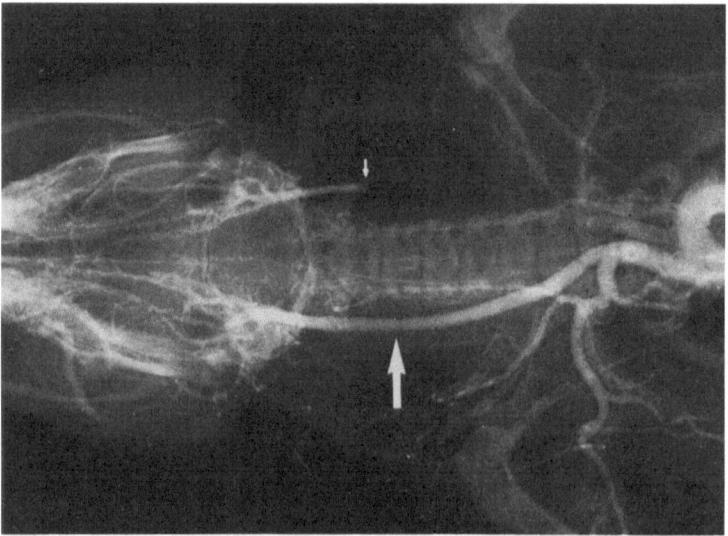

Figs. 23. End-in-end anastomoses on the common carotid artery of the rat. Doppler sonography shows on the right side an acceleration and double peak flow patterns as a sign of a minor to moderate narrowing. On the left side the total flow velocity is reduced because of a severe stenosis with marked local acceleration and unmodulated flow. (Arrows: region of the anastomoses)

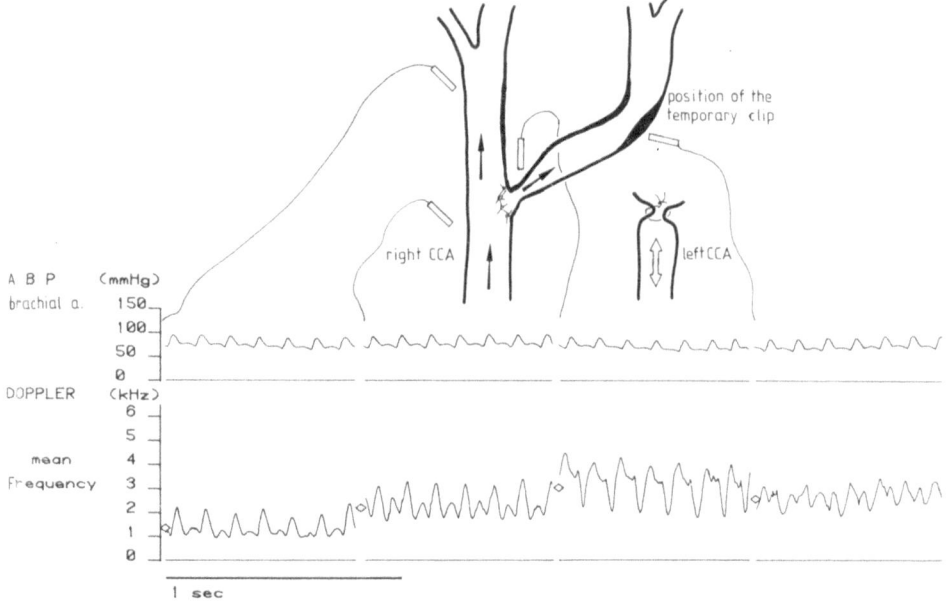

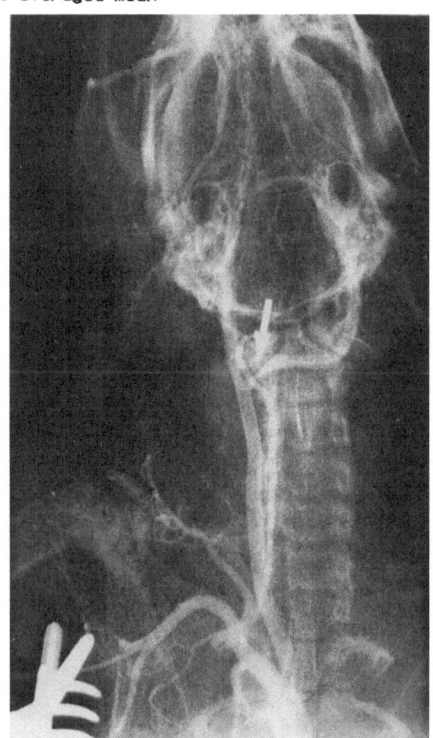

Fig. 24. Classic end-to-side anastomosis with obliquely cut side branch between the right and the distal left common carotid artery of the rat. Doppler sonography shows acceleration and flow irregularities in the distal portion of the anastomosis as a result of narrowing associated with small anastomotic areas. (Arrow: region of the anastomosis with narrowing of the side branch)

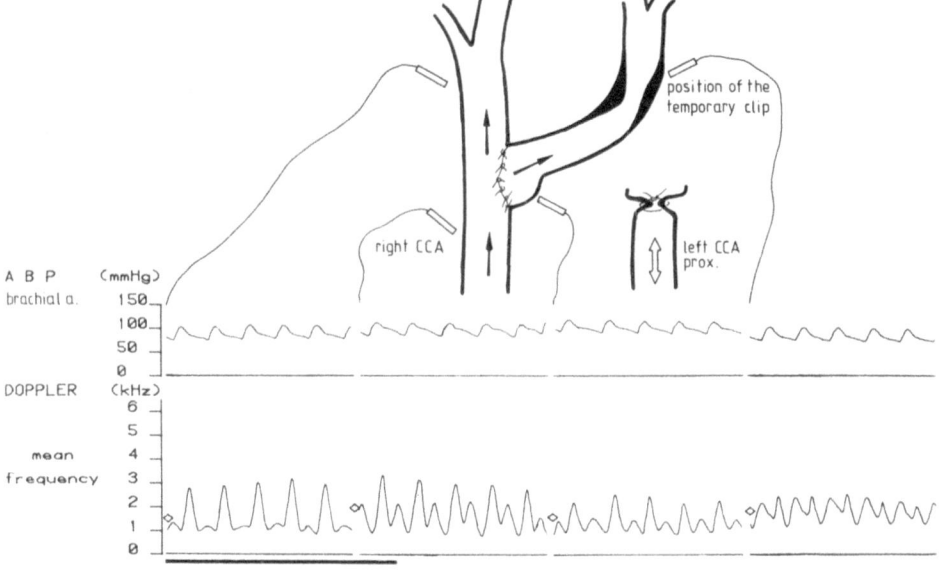

A B P   (mmHg)
brachial a.   150
               100
                50
                 0
DOPPLER   (kHz)
                 6
                 5
    mean   4
frequency   3
                 2
                 1
                 0

o   time averaged mean

Fig. 25. End-to-side anastomoses between the right and the distal left common carotid artery of the rat according to the patch technique. Doppler sonography shows "normal" flow patterns and frequencies in the anastomotic branches and in the area of the anastomosis itself as a sign of a hemodynamically satisfactory anastomosis. Note the acceleration at the site of the temporary clip as a result of vessel wall swelling. (Arrow: region of the anastomosis)

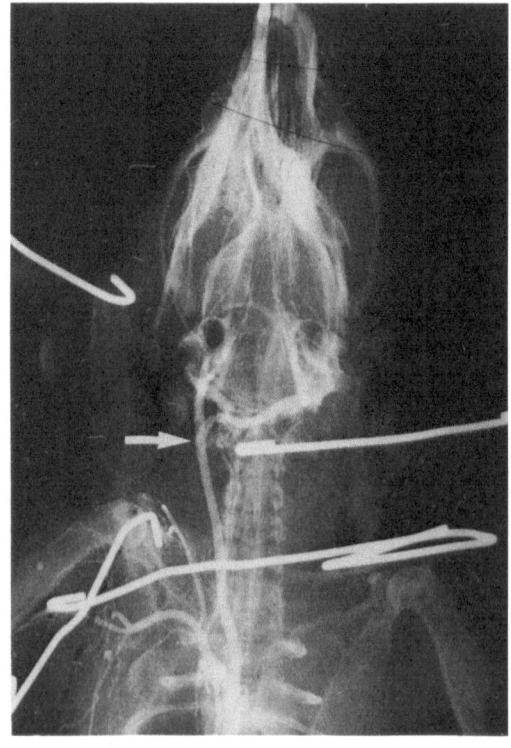

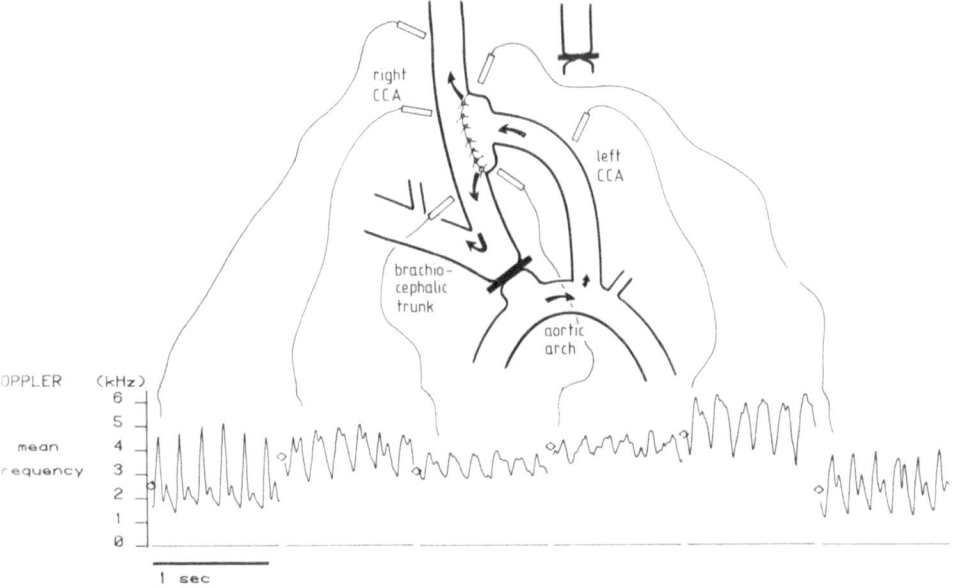

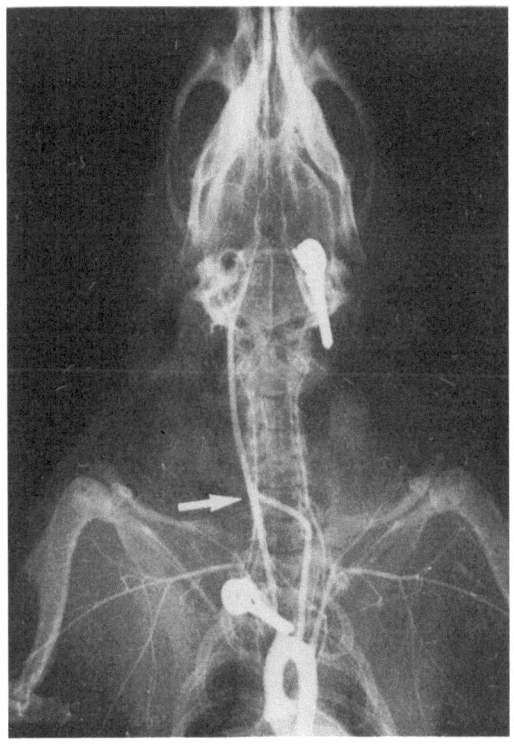

Fig. 26. End-to-side anastomosis between the right common carotid artery and the left proximal carotid artery. The brachiocephalic trunk is clipped to achieve a flow division in the recipient artery similar to extra-intracranial bypass operations. High, but regular Doppler flow pattern in all branches of the anastomosis including the suture area itself. (Arrow: region of the anastomosis)

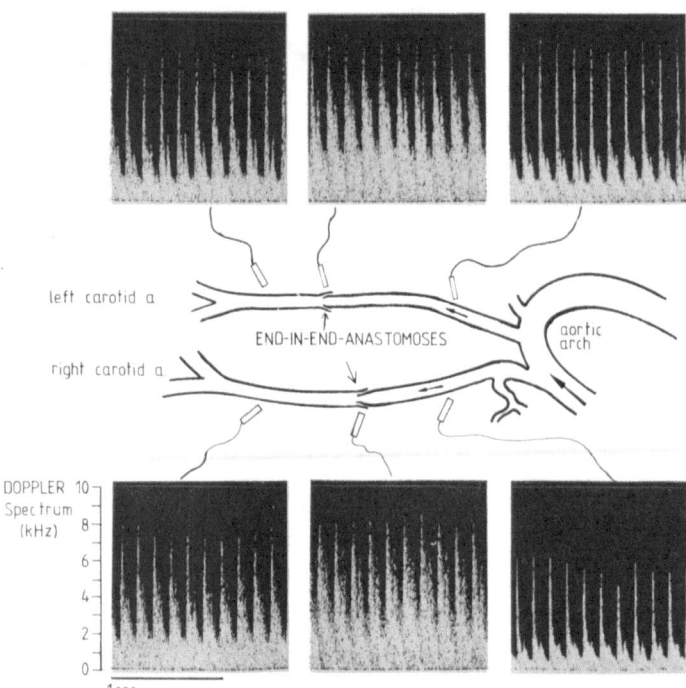

Fig. 27

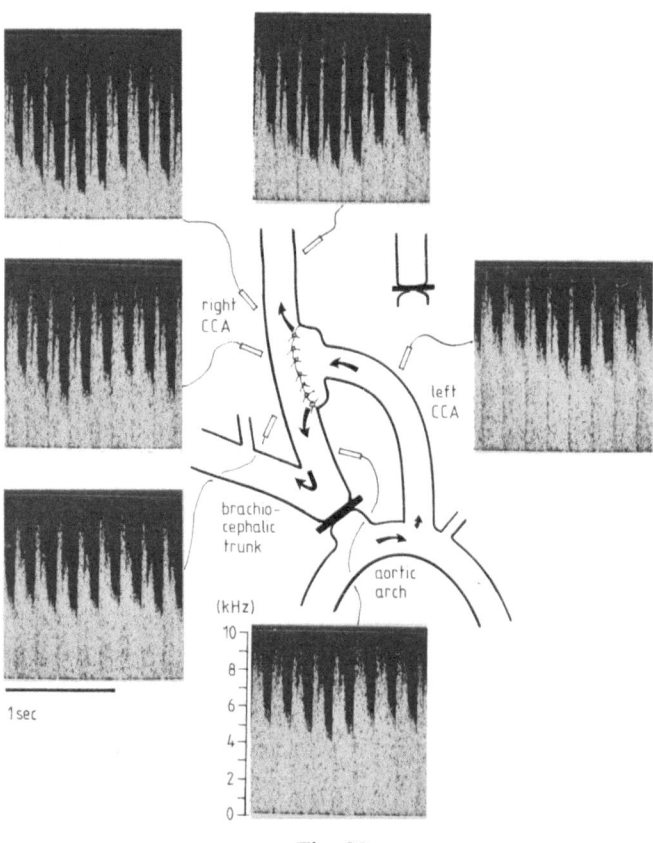

Fig. 28

Figs. 27 and 28. Spectrograms of well functioning end-in-end and end-to-side anastomoses with regular, undisturbed flow and high velocities without marked local acceleration

In the model with left sided main stem and bidirectional flow distribution, the flow usually shows a preference for the brachiocephalic trunk. The hemodynamics in the anastomotic area are similar to the findings in extra-intracranial bypass surgery and are dependent on the suture technique (Fig. 26 and 28).

Discussion

In contrast to the indirect measurement of circulation and flow, with the use of microvascular Doppler sonography it is possible to carry out detailed and repeatable examination of the anastomotic area with special respect to hemodynamic disturbances. Recordings taken after circulation has been re-established register the phase in which, according to morphological findings, the most narrow conditions prevail[2, 122, 159].

In terms of simplicity, amount of information and reliability, Doppler sonography is superior to other methods:

The electromagnetic method of flow measurement reveals only an overall flow, registers pathological findings only after a lumen area reduction of over 80 %, and cannot be used to measure the end-to-side anastomosis itself. The angiographical method, with its unilateral view, only yields valid results if there is a circular stenosis or orthograde imaging of the narrowing.

The stenoses associated with end-to-end anastomoses determined by Doppler sonography confirm the morphological and hemodynamic studies which reveal that narrowings are common among microanastomoses[21, 122, 138, 159, 198]. With regard to end-in-end anastomoses, however, there does not seem to be the same stenosis rate, at least in early investigations[97, 103], but rather a higher stenosis rate as in end-to-end anastomoses[197, 198].

Other than ours, there have been no Doppler sonographic studies reported on experimental end-to-side anastomoses. Our findings have been confirmed by the morphological results of Robertson and Robertson[157], which show that the quality of the anastomosis depends on the number of knots or the surface of the anastomosis. Correspondingly, it can be determined that the large-surface anastomosis according to the patch technique is superior to the diagonal anastomosis.

Conclusions

Using microvascular Doppler sonography, microvascular experimental anastomoses can be examined simply and reliably. Not only the patency, the direction of flow, and the velocity of flow can be studied, but also the local hemodynamic changes in the area of the anastomosis. In this way the quality of an anastomosis can be determined. Stenoses at the site of the anastomosis with corresponding acceleration are to be expected with end-to-end and end-in-end anastomoses. This also holds true for end-to-side anastomoses with oblique incision of the lateral branch. A nearly normal flow is only to be expected with patch anastomoses.

Extracranial-Intracranial Bypass

Introduction

The transcutaneous pre- and postoperative Doppler sono-graphic study of cervical vessels [26, 172] and the postoperative control of the patency and the flow of the extra-intracranial anastomosis [6, 24, 124] are standard examination techniques for occlusive diseases. Intraoperatively, the method is used transcutaneously to localize the donor artery [86, 124, 174, 187] and also to test the patency and to measure flow [126].

There is very little reference in the literature to the branches of the anastomosis [77, 124, 187, 191].

This is due to the lack of commercially available equipment suitable for use on microvessels. Neither electromagnetic flow measurement [39, 46, 85, 162, 173, 174, 179], cerebral blood flow measurement with Xenon [105], the thermodilution method [34] nor the fluorescein angiography [105] have become accepted for routine use.

Microvascular Doppler sonography permits examination of all the essential parts of the extracranial-intracranial anastomoses at the critical point in time — during the operation.

Cases Studied

The study is based on detailed Doppler sonographic measurements of 30 extracranial-intracranial anastomoses between the superficial temporal artery and a branch of the middle cerebral artery in cases of occlusions and stenoses of the cervical or cavernous internal carotid artery. The reasons for surgery were transitory ischemic attacks, strokes and asymptomatic carotid artery occlusions prior to scheduled aorto-coronary bypass surgery.

Methods

The same anastomotic technique was used in all cases: an infrasylvian branch of the middle cerebral artery was sought out under an osteoplastic trepanation approximately 6 cm above the auditory canal. This branch was connected mostly to the parietal branch of the superficial temporal artery following the patch technique[3, 158].

For the routine examination the following examination procedure has proved to be useful and efficient (Table 2):

Table 2. *Doppler ultrasonic examination procedure during extracranial-intracranial bypass operation*

vessel studied	information/reason for study
superficial temporal artery	course of artery and its branches, participation of frontal branch on ophthalmic collateral flow
skin supplying frontal branch, dissected	participation on ophthalmic collateral flow
skin supplying parietal (donor) branch, dissected	"normal" and control value
donor branch, distal cut	maximum flow volume and velocity, basal value for computing anastomotic flow
recipient vessel before anastomosis	flow direction for anastomosis direction and identification of Sylvian fissure, basal value for anastomotic flow distribution
distal donor artery after anastomosis	patency, anastomotic flow volume by velocity comparison
donor artery at site of clips	stenoses dure to temporary clip
distal/proximal recipient vessel after anastomosis	patency, flow change, flow distribution, stenoses by temporary clips
anastomosis area	flow impairment, irregularities
donor artery before wound closure	secondary thrombosis, kinking

The measurements can be taken with the probe in direct contact with the vessels. There is sufficient room to obtain the optimum probe angle (approx. 50 degrees) for the Doppler signal. The entire crossection can be covered with the 0.7 and the 1.3 mm gate width, so that the Doppler frequency corresponds to the mean velocity in the entire vessel.

Transcutaneous Intraoperative Measurements of the Donor Artery

The small ultrasonic beam and the high resolution even with vessels measured in millimeters, make it possible to plot precisely the course of the superficial temporal artery with its branches. By this mapping, the dissection of the temporal artery is facilitated and accelerated, particularly if longitudinal sections are used (Fig. 29).

A retrograde flow in the supratrochlear artery and high diastolic flow with a low resistance index in the frontal branch signifies participation in ophthalmical collateralization. Thus the frontal branch can be considered as a donor artery only in exceptional cases (Fig. 30). The mean Doppler frequencies of the normal temporal artery were 0.2—1.8 kHz (average 1 kHz) with a resistance index of 0.8 (0.7—1.0), which is typical for the external arterial system (Figs. 30, 42 and 43).

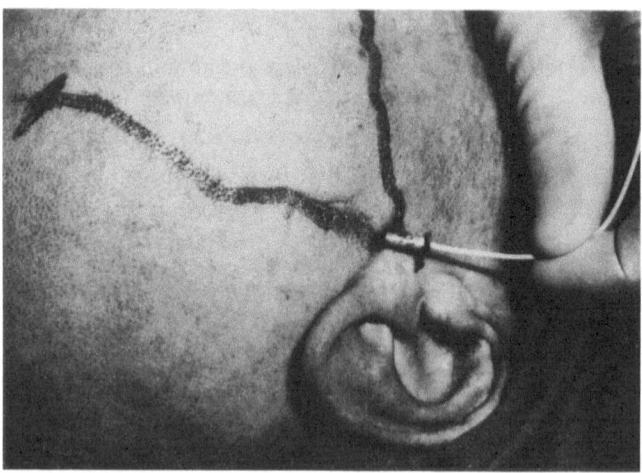

Fig. 29. Transcutaneous Doppler mapping of the course of the donor artery (superficial temporal artery) with its branches (frontal and parietal ramus)

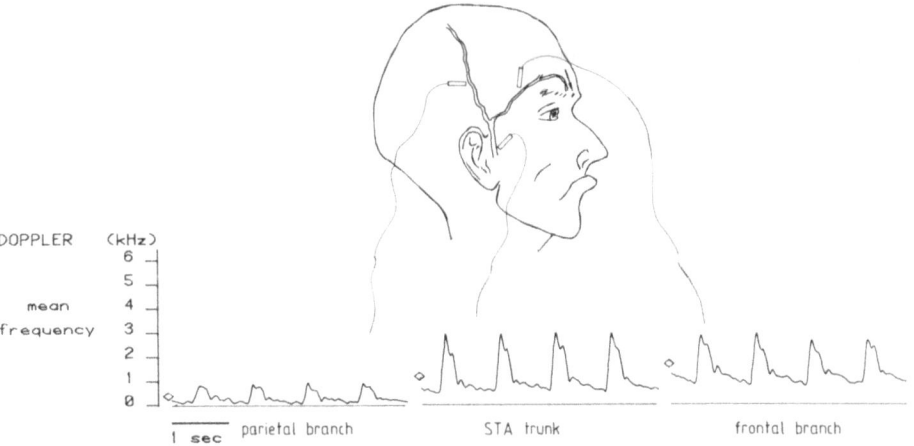

o: time averaged mean

Fig. 30. Flow pattern of the superficial temporal artery with its branches during intraoperative transcutaneous measuring before anastomosis. Note the high diastolic flow in the main stem and in the frontal branch which signifies participation in ophthalmic collateral flow with retrograde flow in the supratrochlear artery

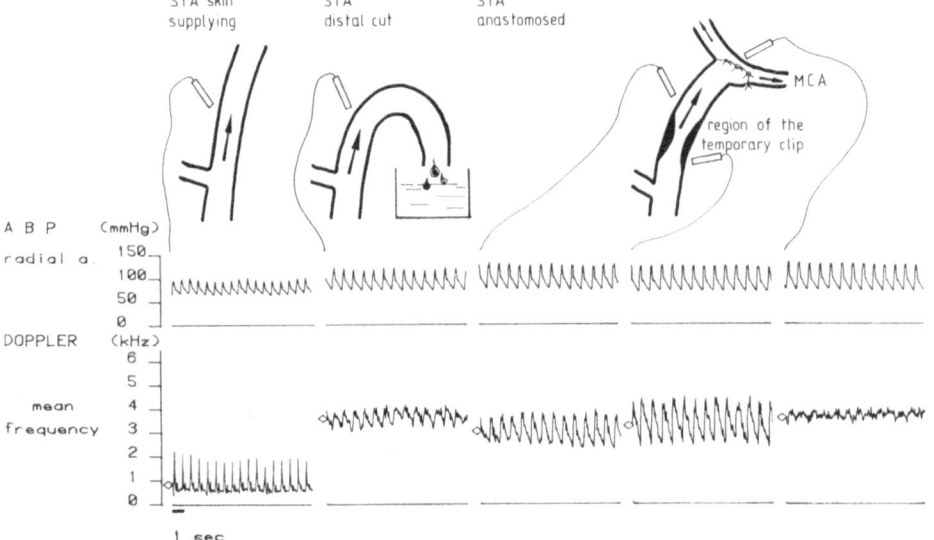

o: time averaged mean

Fig. 31. Typical flow pattern during direct measurement of the superficial temporal artery before and after being cut and after being connected to the cerebral vascular system

Direct Measurements of the Donor Artery Before Anastomosis

To determine the approximate flow of the anastomosed donor artery by comparing velocities, the Doppler frequency in the open temporal artery has to be determined as well as the blood volume, which is collected in a pot (Figs. 31 and 38).

For the separated temporal artery, volumina of 6—60 ccm, average 25 ccm, can be expected, depending on blood pressure, caliber, and transverse section of the distal end. The Doppler frequencies range between 1—4.4 kHz (average 3 kHz).

Measurement of Recipient Artery Before Anastomosis

The Doppler sonographic determination of the direction of the recipient vessel can be helpful in identifying the Sylvian fissure and in determining the direction of the anastomosis, which should be towards the fissure where the greatest requirement is. With a choice of several possible recipient vessels of the same size, the vessel having the slowest flow should be selected.

In the examined cases of cervical occlusion of the carotid arteries, the flow in the middle cerebral artery branches was orthograde. The mean Doppler frequencies were between 0.3 and 2.0 kHz (average 0.9 kHz) in vessels with an outer diameter of 0.8—2.0 mm (Figs. 32 and 38). Frequencies over 0.8 kHz with the same transverse section were found in patients with healthy vessels who were operated on for other reasons.

Extremely slow velocities resembling venous flow with weak pulsations are typical for patients with multiple arterial occlusions (Fig. 32). Normal flow curves and velocities are observed only in patients with unilateral carotid occlusion or stenosis.

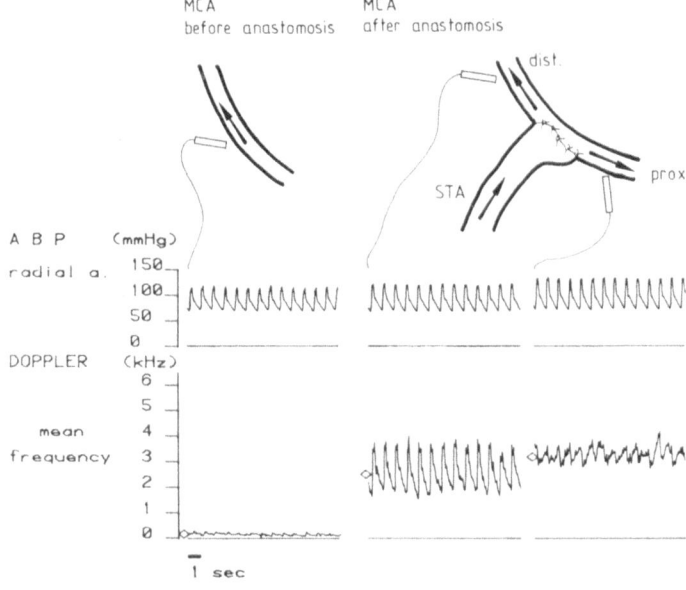

Fig. 32. Typical flow pattern of the recipient branch of the middle cerebral artery. Note the slightly modulated almost vein-like flow before anastomosis and the high almost turbulent retrograde flow after anastomosis

Findings Among Normal Anastomoses

After the anastomosis has been completed and circulation re-established, the temporal artery is examined to see whether the anastomotic flow is functioning and, if so, if flow is in the desired direction. If these findings are satisfactory, the critical points are checked for irregularities and flow acceleration, i. e., the site of the temporary clip on the donor artery, the anastomotic area itself, particularly the acute-angled portion and the proximal and distal branches of the recipient artery (Figs. 31, 32, 33 and 39).

The measurements taken on the donor artery of a hemodynamically effective anastomosis show the typical change from the so-called external to inernal type, i. e., besides an increase in the mean flow velocity, there is above all a relative increase in the diastolic flow with a corresponding decrease in the resistance index (Figs. 31 and 33). The mean

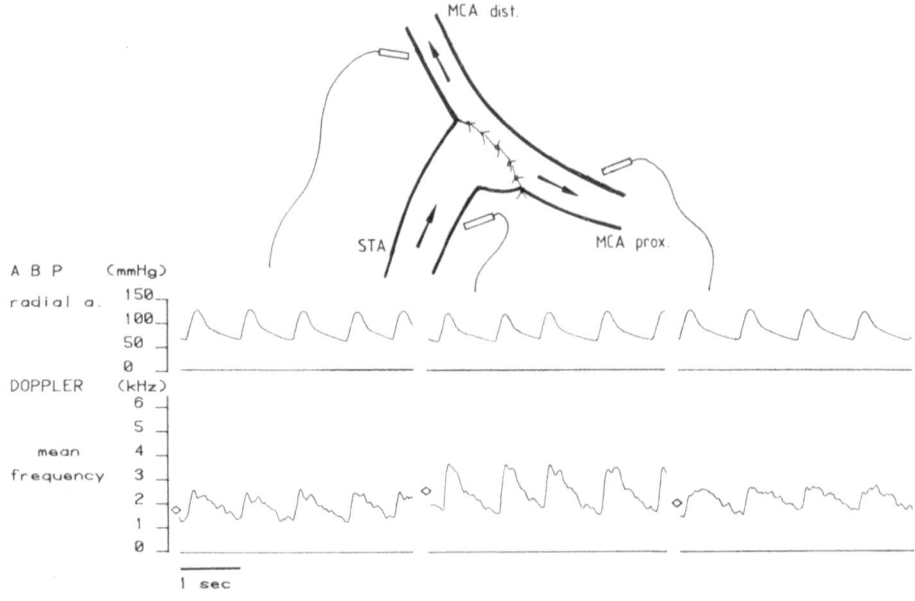

Fig. 33. Flow pattern of a well-functioning anastomosis

Doppler frequencies are 1.5—4.4 kHz (average 2.8 kHz) and can be 1—7 times (average 3.4 times) higher than those of the skin supplying donor artery. An increase in the velocity of the anastomosed donor artery, in comparison to the open donor artery, can also occur if no sufficient vessel stump paralysis is achieved during the first measurements (in 50 % of our cases).

The flow, which can be calculated approximately according to the method of Mueller and Gratzl[126] by comparing the flow velocities of the open and of the anastomosed temporal arteries, was in our cases between 5 and 55 ccm/min (average 23.2 ccm/min).

Almost without exception (29 out of 30 cases) an anastomosis flows bidirectionally: distally in the original direction and proximally towards the Sylvian fissure where there is flow reversal (Figs. 33 and 39) type-T distribution.

Only exceptionally (1 out of 30 cases) the bypass takes part solely in the distal flow, type-L distribution (Figs. 34 and 46). Apart from hemodynamic reasons (see chapter on controlled carotid ligation) a mechanical impediment always has to be considered as the cause in these cases.

In the type-T flow distribution, the flow towards the fissure is predominant. The retrograde flow velocity is on the average five time higher (1—15 times) than the originally orthograde velocity. The flow velocity in the distal branch of the anastomosis is also about four times higher (1—10 times) than before anastomosis.

The mean Doppler frequencies obtainable from the proximal portion of the anastomosed middle cerebral artery branch range between 0.8 and 4.6 kHz (average 2.5 kHz) and from the distal part between 0.8 and 3.2 kHz (average 1.9 kHz). The resistance index in the recipient artery distal to the anastomosis has approximately the same value (0.17—0.79, average 0.49) as the recipient vessel before anastomosis (0.27—0.6, average 0.47). The proximal branch, however, shows a marked reduction (0.17—0.67, average 0.39).

In the 30 anastomoses examined, the last measurement taken in the suture area before closing the wound showed a laminar flow. Only exceptionally were accelerations observed at the acute-angled part or flow irregularities at the obtuse-angled part.

Pathological Findings in Anastomoses

In about 10 % (in our material 3 out of 30 cases) occlusions can be expected intraoperatively, although this is not apparent from the external appearance of the sutures. The absence of the Doppler signal or a "dead end" signal provides unambiguous recognition of the occlusion. In our experience there is a risk of thrombosis between the site of the temporary clip on the donor artery and the anastomosis (Figs. 34 and 40). The recipient artery may, however, remain open in this case, but with an orthograde, and in some cases, diminished, flow in the proximal branch in comparison to before anastomosis (Fig. 35). In such cases, one must act immediately to reopen the anastomosis partially, in order to flush out the vessel, so as to ensure the function of the anastomosis. In the three cases treated in this way, the anastomosis remained open (Figs. 36 and 41).

Stenoses can occur at the acute-angled portion of the anastomosis itself, as shown in two cases (7 %). If hemodynamically effective, they can be detected through a flow velocity reduction distal to the stenosis; if not, only local accelerations or irregularities are present. In the cases of subtotal occlusion, milking may be effective, as shown by our cases. In the recipient artery itself neither thrombosis nor stenosis are observed.

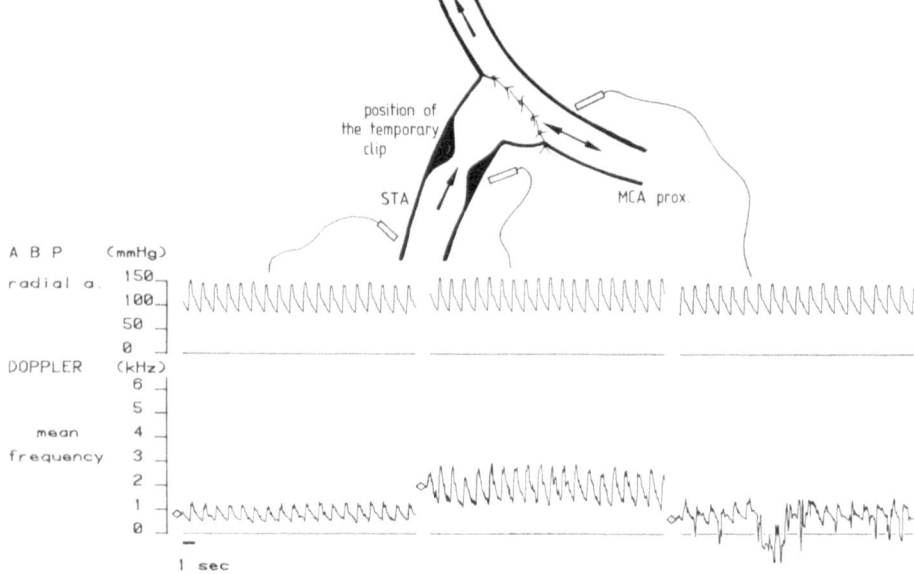

o: time averaged mean

Fig. 34. Flow pattern of the donor and proximal recipient artery in an unsatisfactory anastomosis. Note the lack of a clear retrograde flow in the proximal middle cerebral artery branch and the slow flow in the temporal artery with a marked acceleration in the region of the temporary clip. This anastomosis thrombosed intraoperatively (Fig. 35) and had to be reopened

Fig. 35. Flow pattern of an anastomosis with donor artery occlusion. Note the orthograde slow flow in the recipient vessel as before anastomosis (Fig. 32) and the absence of retrograde flow in the proximal portion of the recipient artery

Fig. 36. Procedure in a case of donor artery occlusion: partial reopening of the suture, milking of the artery in order to remove clots and to restore the flow; elevation of the blood pressure and — most effective — irrigation with heparin solution

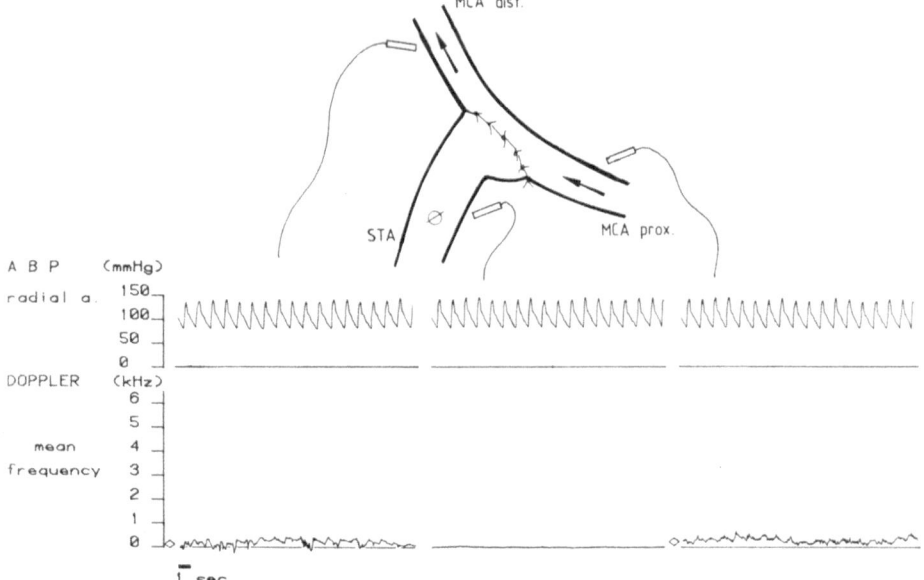

Fig. 35

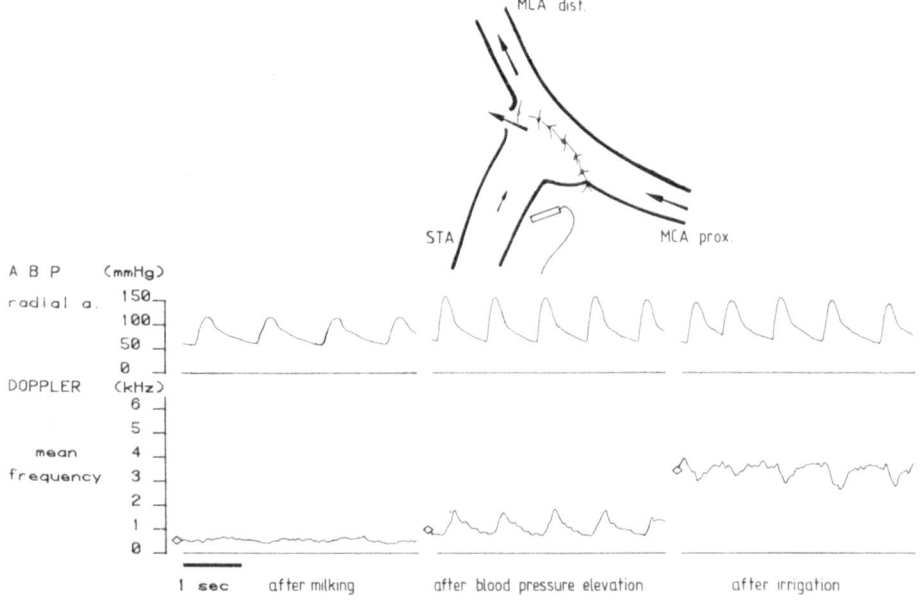

Fig. 36

Postoperative Transcutaneous Measurements

The intraoperative Doppler velocity meter is also useful for postoperative patency control. Sure signs of a patent anastomosis include: a Doppler frequency of the donor artery that is more than twice that of the opposite side and of the measurment taken preoperatively, a reduction in the resistance index from the external to the internal type, a temporal artery that can be followed almost to the trepanation, and a lasting flow during compression of the non-participating branch (Figs. 37 and 43).

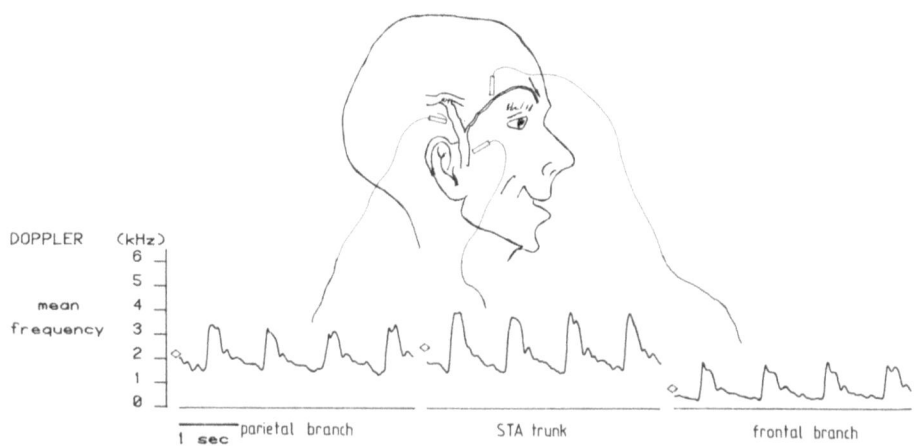

o: time averaged mean

Fig. 37. Flow pattern of the superficial temporal artery with its branches during postoperative transcutaneous control of a functioning anastomosis. Note the high diastolic flow (internal type) in the donor artery (parietal branch of the STA) with reduced flow in the frontal branch in comparison with pre-operative measurements

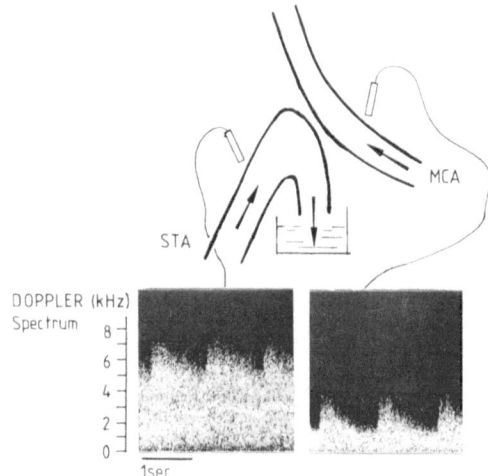

Fig. 38. Basic values of the two bypass parts: maximum flow velocity and volume of the donor artery, original orthograde flow in the recipient artery

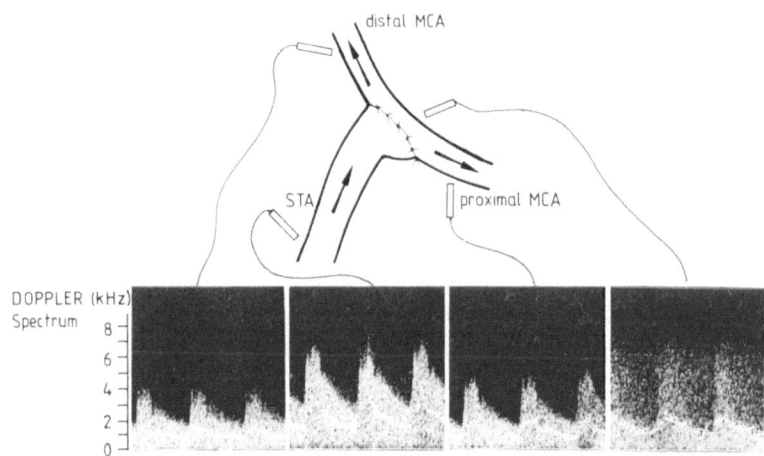

Fig. 39. Findings in a well-functioning anastomosis with a high, undisturbed flow in all components and only slight irregularities in the anastomotic area itself

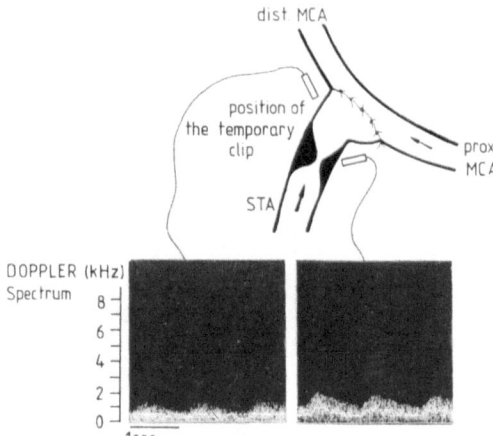

Fig. 40. Findings in a high grade stenosis of the donor artery with very slow flow and weak acceleration in the region of the temporary clip

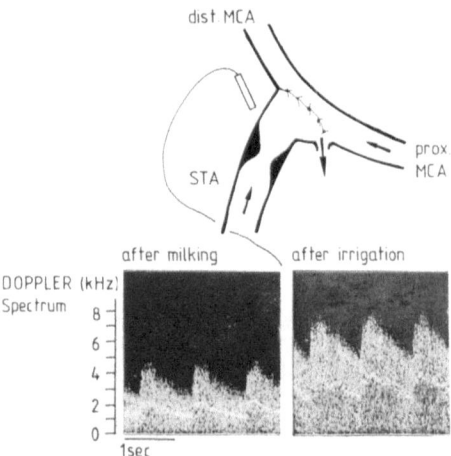

Fig. 41. Treatment of an occlusion of the donor artery with partial re-opening of the suture, milking and irrigation

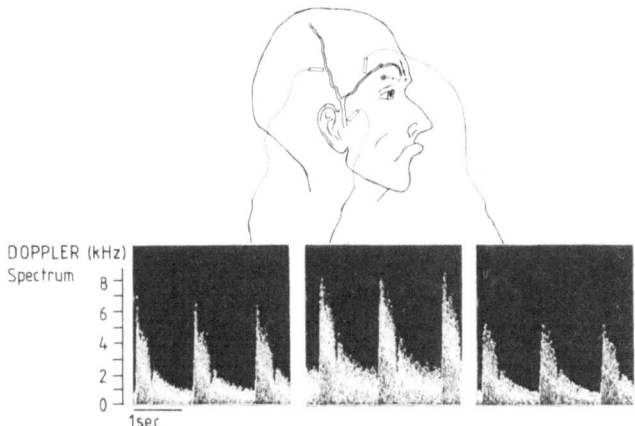

Fig. 42

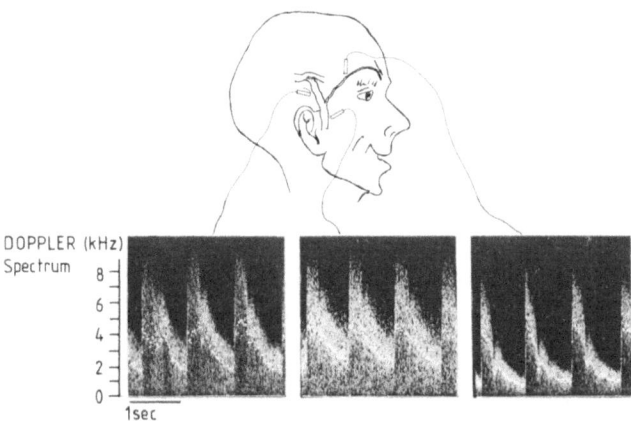

Fig. 43

Figs. 42 and 43. Transcutaneous findings before (42) and after (43) anastomosis. Note the elevation of the entire velocity with a relatively high diastolic component in the donor artery

Discussion

There are no definitive conclusions in the literature as to when and why anastomotic occlusions occur in up to 10 % of cases. However, some findings, including those of Little et al.[105], who detected intraoperative occlusions using fluorescein angiography, animal experiments of Rosenbaum and Sundt[159], and our own results with 3 out of 30 intraoperative anastomotic occlusions, seem to indicate that the decisive point in time for the fate of an anastomosis is between the removal of the temporary clips and the closure of the incision. Reliable intraoperative methods to test anastomotic patency and to rule out stenoses, which are a potential risk of secondary occlusion, are therefore important for the success of the operation. Methods such as the simple inspection of the anastomosis[1] and the unnecessarily traumatizing mechanical patency test[1, 47, 79] can at the most provide information that there is a flow, but neither the direction nor the strength, and are thus outdated by electronic test methods.

The electromagnetic technique of flow measurement, which due to anatomic factors can be applied only in the area of the donor artery, usually provides precise information on flow direction and intensity for an exposed area only. Information on the quality of the anastomosis is unreliable since the various pressure conditions in the internal and external arterial system make it difficult to estimate what flow is normal for amounts varying from 93—10 ccm[85, 173]. Furthermore, for hemodynamic reasons even a normal flow for the individual case does not rule out lumen stenoses of up to 80 %[19].

Intraoperative regional measurements of cerebral blood flow with the Xenon or the thermodilution methods only yield information on the functioning bypass, provided there is an increase in the cerebral flow. They provide no information, however, on the quality of the anastomosis. The same limitations apply to fluorescein angiography, which can reveal flow changes in the visible cortical vessels before and after bypass.

The microvascular Doppler technique, in contrast, is an atraumatic and repeatable method of examining the anastomosis itself and every point of the three anastomotic branches. Flow impairment can be detected from a

cross-section area reduction of 40 % upwards, i.e., long before a hemodynamic effect is detectable. This method thus
not only helps to determine the patency and the flow direction, but is also an aid in producing qualitatively well-functioning anastomoses. In cases of occlusion or stenosis, limited treatment is possible because of the known site of impairment.

There is little known about the hemodynamics of the cortical middle cerebral arteries as potential recipient vessels.
Studies using fluorescein angiography have revealed that occlusive disease causes an extension of the cortical transit
times [105] and blood pressure measurements taken with the
puncture method [41, 66, 85, 123, 180, 204] have shown that pressure is
lower among patients with occlusive disease than in patients
without [10, 202]. Flow velocity and flow volume have hardly
been examined. Doppler examinations of cortical recipient
arteries in patients with occlusive disease have only been
carried out by Moritake et al. [124]. Among 15 patients, they
studied 17 cortical recipient vessels and found no flow in 5
cases, poor orthograde flow in 9 cases, and good orthograde
flow in 3 cases. The arteries showing no flow were not
closed, since they served as recipient vessels. The reason for
the lack of flow detectability can be attributed to the equipment used, which was not suited for small vessels and low
velocities.

The reduction of flow volume of the anastomosed temporal artery, in comparison to the open artery, as reported
by Spetzler and Chater [173] was observed in less than half of
our patients. The reason for this discrepancy, since the maximum flow capacity was about the same, could be the lack of
vessel stump paralysis as well as a different anastomotic
technique with a higher degree of permeability.

The anastomosed temporal arteries examined by Doppler
sonography always had a measurable flow in comparison to
those measured electromagnetically, provided there was patency. The fact that Moritake et al. [124] were unable to detect
flow, even though patency was established by angiography
after the operation, must be due to the measuring technique
and not to an occlusion.

Intraoperative studies on the distribution of the anastomotic flow were carried out only by Moritake et al. [124]. They
reported bilateral blood flow in 44 % and a purely peripheral

flow in 56 % of their cases. These results are surprising when one considers that the cases studied were similar to ours and cannot be attributed to the measuring technique. They are also contradicted by the usual findings of postoperative angiographical follow-ups, which indicate that bilateral flow distribution is evident in more than 90 % of the cases [102, 188].

All intraoperatively observed thromboses occurred in the donor artery between the temporary clip and the anastomosis. In comparison, Little et al. [105] reported one such case from among 15 anastomoses. These thromboses demonstrate how the relatively strong clips placed proximal to the anastomosis endanger the temporarily cut-off donor artery, which is void of blood flow over a considerable length. A peripherally placed clip with a low pressure gradient thus seems more advisable.

The direct intraoperative Doppler measurements show that, as in animal experiments, the patch technique is hemodynamically ideal for bypass operations also in man.

Conclusions

Thromboses and stenoses after extracranial-intracranial anastomoses mostly occur intraoperatively. They are not visible externally and must be measured by Doppler sonography. Predominantly affected are the donor artery and the acute-angled portion of the anastomotic area. An absence of flow in the donor artery or the lack of an increase in flow velocity in the recipient artery indicate the need for revision of the anastomoses.

The criteria for a hemodynamically efficient anastomosis are: 1) Flow velocity of the donor artery must be at least the same or higher than that of the skin-supplying artery, with a significantly reduced resistance index. 2) No acceleration in the area of the temporary clips. 3) Laminar flow at the anastomosis, or at the most, slight irregularities and acceleration at the acute angle. 4) Flow distribution towards the fissure as well as distal to the anastomosis. 5) In the recipient artery distal flow velocity at least the same or higher and proximal in the reversed direction with equal or greater velocity.

Bypass for Giant Aneurysms

Introduction

In the treatment of giant aneurysms by carotid ligation and simultaneous extracranial-intracranial bypass, there are various opinions as to when the cervical internal carotid artery should be occluded: immediately after the bypass has been completed[82], one day later[143], within 1—2 days[69], within 2—3 days[23, 174], or within 7—10 days[48]. What is agreed, however, is that a high pressure gradient in the area of the anastomosis is desirable, i. e., a reduction of the carotid flow is aimed for from the start.

If the carotid artery is occluded before the bypass has adequately functioned, there is a risk of ischemic complications[23, 69]. If the carotid flow is maintained too long, thrombus formation from the aneurysm can lead to embolic complications[48, 118].

The risk of ischemic complications in carotid ligation can be lowered by pre- or intraoperative measurement of the cerebral blood flow with temporarily occluded carotid artery[69, 143], by measuring the stump pressure of the cervical internal carotid artery[23, 174], and by detailed angiographic studies. However, the risk cannot be ruled out entirely[23, 69].

Intraoperative Doppler sonography makes it possible to carry out controlled carotid narrowing suitable for the anastomosis by taking measurements directly in the area of the anastomosis.

Cases Studied

The findings presented are based on three patients with giant aneurysms in the cavernous part of the carotid artery.

They were treated by cervical carotid ligation and simultaneous extra-intracranial bypass between the superficial temporal artery and a branch of the middle cerebral artery.

Cervical Measurements

The critical number of turns of the Selverstone clamp under which reduction of the blood flow in the internal carotid artery commences is first obtained by taking Doppler measurements distal to the clamp while the artery is progressively occluded. Experience has confirmed that a reduction of flow velocity does not occur until the clamp has been turned 6—7 times, whereas 8 times will occlude the artery (Fig. 44).

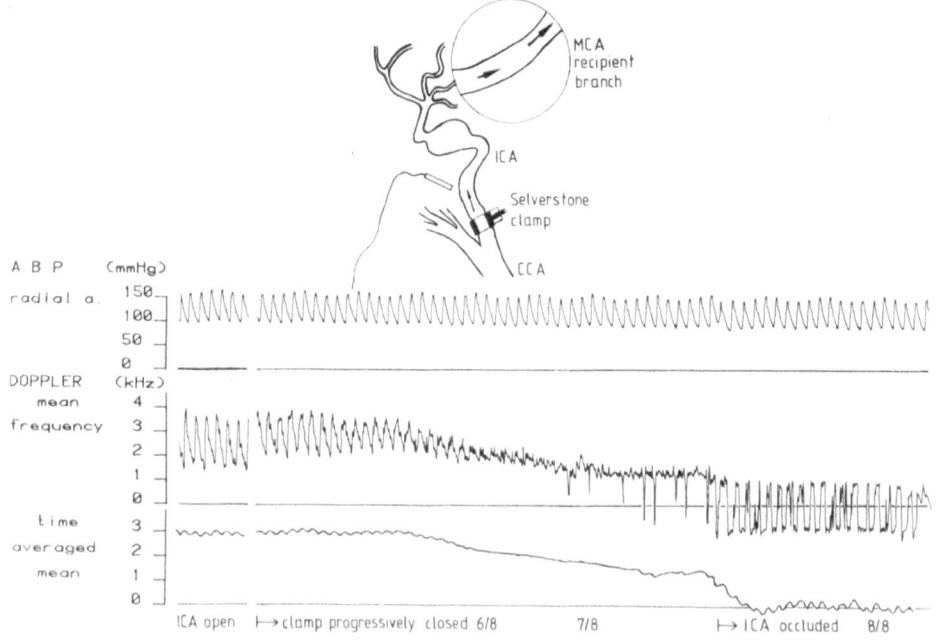

Fig. 44. Flow pattern of the cervical internal carotid artery with progressively closed Selverstone clamp. Note that the flow velocity reduction begins only in high grade stenosis and the "dead end" pulse pattern after complete occlusion

Intracranial Measurements Before Anastomosis

Change of the blood flow velocity in a not yet dissected recipient vessel with simultaneously performed carotid ligation to the point of occlusion gives information on the hemodynamic consequences of carotid ligation without bypass. In each of the three cases, a reduction of the mean flow velocity and of the amplitude modulation to a minimum of 30 % of the original value was observed. In each case the orthograde flow direction remained unchanged (Fig. 45).

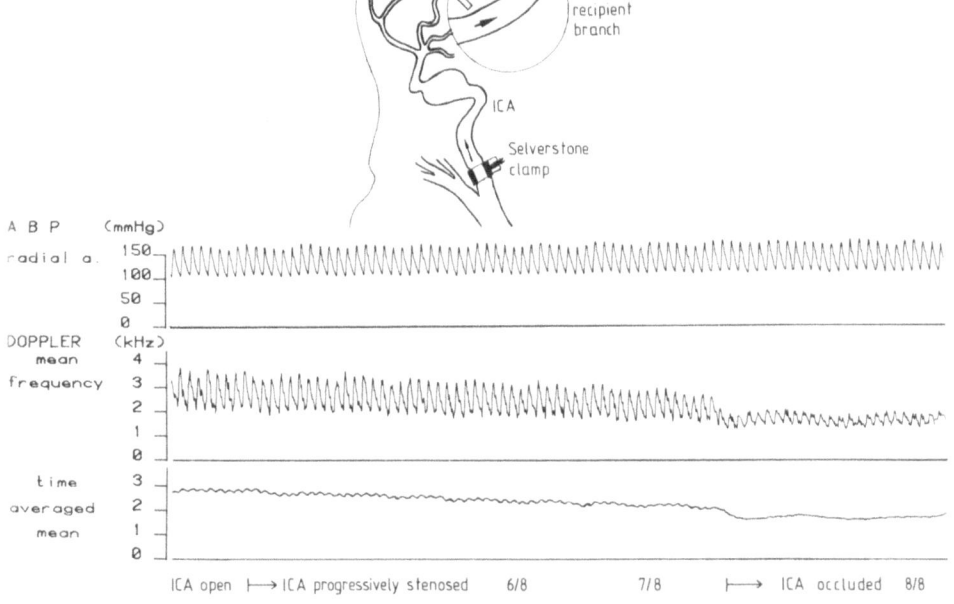

Fig. 45. Flow pattern of the recipient middle cerebral artery branch before anastomosis with patent and progressively closed cervical internal carotid artery. Note the good orthograde flow velocity after complete internal carotid occlusion

Intracranial Measurements After Anastomosis

Apart from the routine measurements, special attention is paid to the branch proximal to the anastomosis during staged carotid ligation. This is because a retrograde flow towards the fissure signifies a well-functioning anastomosis.

In 2 of the 3 cases, an "alternating flow" could be observed in the branch proximal to the anastomosis, which turned to a clearly retrograde flow after the cervical carotid artery was subtotally ligated. The third case showed an extremely slow retrograde filling of the proximal branch, which clearly increased as the carotid artery was stenosed (Fig. 46).

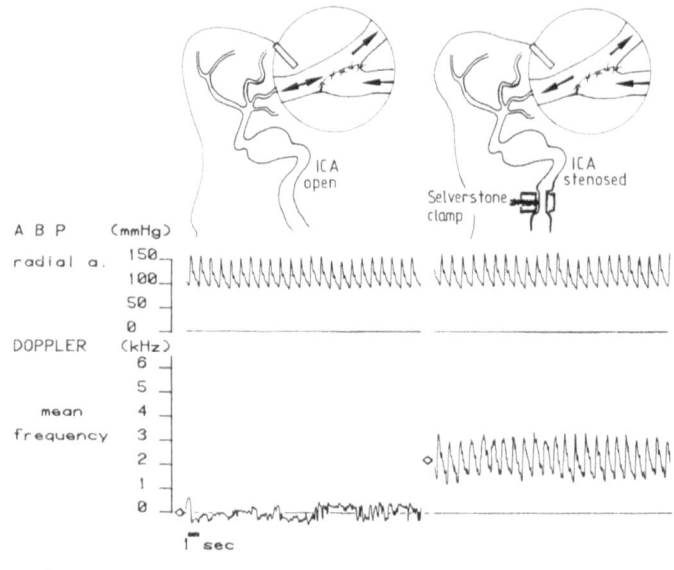

Fig. 46. Flow pattern in the recipient artery proximal to the anastomosis: on the left with carotid artery open, on the right with subtotal carotid ligation. The alternating flow on the left is due to the equal pressure in the external and internal arterial system; the retrograde flow starts after lowering the internal pressure by turning the Selverstone clamp on the internal carotid artery

Postoperative Transcutaneous Measurement

If the postoperative transcutaneous follow-up reveals a sustained properly functioning anastomotic flow, which increases even more while the carotid artery is temporarily occluded, the artery can then be occluded permanently.

Discussion

The Doppler ultrasound examination of a cortical middle cerebral artery branch during staged ligation of the internal carotid artery, which has already been referred to by Moritake et al.[124], is of use only at the time of the operation and for the orthograde blood flow in the circulation area of the vessel under investigation. A reduction of the perfusion of the middle cerebral artery is, however, a measure for the hemodynamic effect which, in the most unfavourable cases, can lead to neurological deficits from the lack of collateral compensation. If one assumes that a reduction of the cerebral blood flow to one third causes deficiency symptoms[69, 184], a decrease in flow velocity beyond that point has to be considered dangerous. Correspondingly, no significant ischemic complications were expected in our own cases, even without bypass.

Besides judging the risk of ischemic complications, the second problem is producing adequate bypass flow. This means that there must be a sufficient pressure gradient between the external and internal circulation. That this is not always the case has been proved by 2 of 13 cases reported by Spetzler et al.[174], which had an intracranial-extracranial flow. Since the patency of anastomosis depends on a great as possible flow in all sections, the hemodynamics in the anastomotic area have to be the measure for adequate carotid ligation. Ligating the carotid artery by approximately 50 % by pressure or flow measurements taken in the cervical area[48, 174], which up till now has been the common procedure, is by comparison less precise and less specific.

Conclusions

Doppler measurements at the site of anastomosis in controlled narrowing of the cervical carotid artery until the onset of an adequate flow produce the best prerequisite for a well functioning bypass and reduces the risk of ischemia due to unnecessarily high grade stenosis.

Aneurysms

Introduction

Despite the favorable conditions of microsurgery, occlusion or stenosis of supplying or neighboring vessels which are neither intended nor detectable can occur during aneurysm clipping[91, 107, 186, 193]. Incomplete clipping, which poses the risk of postoperative bleeding, is also possible[53, 186].

Such complications could be immediately corrected if angiography were performed intraoperatively[109, 142, 199]. However, for technical reasons, this method has not been adopted. Instead, angiography is recommended directly after the operation[193].

Electromagnetic flow measuring[131, 132] can only be done on individual vessels and is hardly conductive to controlling surgical measures.

Doppler sonography has up to now only been used by Nornes et al.[134, 135] to assess the patency of the supplying vessels and to control aneurysm clipping. However, for known reasons of equipment limitations, the Doppler method has not yet been generally adopted.

The microvascular Doppler system, because of its small probe sizes and measuring range, offers the best prerequisite for carrying out useful measurements during aneurysm surgery at the circle of Willis.

Cases Studied

The findings are based on examinations of more than 250 individual vessels in 50 patients with 53 aneurysms. The aneurysms included: 1 ophthalmic, 7 at the posterior communicating artery, 4 at the bifurcation of the internal carotid artery, 10 at the bifurcation of the middle cerebral artery, 24 of the anterior communicating artery, 5 of the distal anterior cerebral artery, and 2 of the vertebral artery at the origin of the PICA.

Forty-seven aneurysms had hemorrhaged, 6 had been detected for other reasons. In 19 cases, the last subarachnoid hemorrhage had occurred less than 72 hours before, in 16 cases between 4 and 14 days, and in 12 cases more than 14 days prior to operation. The grade of risk, according to the grading scale of Hunt and Hess[83], was between 0 and III. All but 2 aneurysms were clipped under neurolept-anesthesia and under normotension, normocapnia, and normothermia. In 14 patients the blood pressure was temporarily lowered with sodium nitroprusside because of dissection complications or premature rupture. Postoperative angiography was carried out in the first 45 patients under the same surgical anesthesia. After the reliability of the Doppler sonographic examination had been established, angiography was performed only for special indications.

Examination Procedure

The following examination procedure has proved to be useful and efficient for standard aneurysm operations and for special investigations (Table 3):

Table 3. *Routine measurements during aneurysm surgery (upper half) and additional examinations (lower half, see p. 70)*

investigated vessel	reason for investigation/information
parent arteries before clipping	initial findings for pulse curve and velocity comparisons after clipping; spasms after former SAH and hyperemia after recent SAH; spasms caused by dissection
aneurysm after clipping	complete clipping; Doppler controlled clip positioning
parent arteries after clipping	patency; lumen reduction caused by clips, plaques, torison and mechanical spasm

	special reasons for investigation
aneurysm before clipping	distinction of aneurysm from normal brain vessels; partial thrombosis; plaques
brain vessels	effect of topical and systematic vasodilators

If because of cramped conditions the probe cannot be brought into direct contact with the vessels, effective examination can be achieved by filling the cisterns with liquid. Investigations are then possible under visual control through the liquid even over a distance of 2—3 mm. However, more than 90 % of the vessels can be examined directly, although optimal angular adjustment is not always achieved.

The best recordings are achieved with gates of 0.7 and 1.3 mm, which approximately take in the cross-sections of

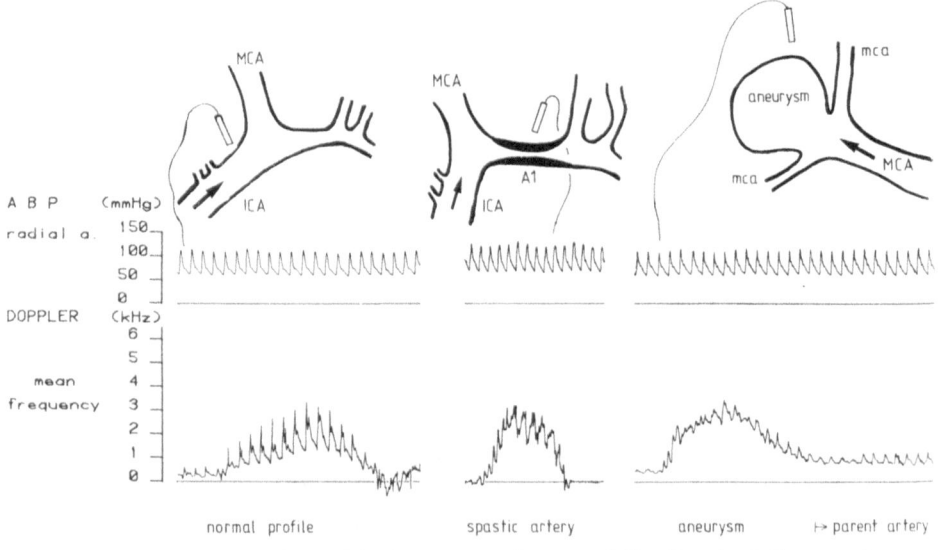

Fig. 47. Flow profiles with the automatic gate shift: On the left normal flat profile of a great intracranial vessel; in the middle a sharp steep profile with pathological flow pulse curves because of acceleration in a spastic artery; on the right flat profile with regular flow patterns in a giant aneurysm

the vessels. The Doppler frequency spectrum is then proportional to the mean velocity of the entire vessel cross-section.
The automatic gate shift of the smallest gate is of use in obtaining an impression of the width of the lumen (Fig. 47).

Normal Flow Pattern

The flow pulse waveforms in the parent arteries are regular
after subarachnoid hemorrhages have subsided or in cases of
aneurysms with no preceding hemorrhaging. They have a
relatively high diastolic flow, an index of resistance of
0.2—0.7 (average 0.53), and mean Doppler frequencies between 0.8 and 6 kHz (Figs. 48 and 49).

Table 4 shows the mean Doppler frequencies measured in
those vessels at the base of the brain which are the most fre-
quent sites of aneurysms. They reveal that the flow velocity

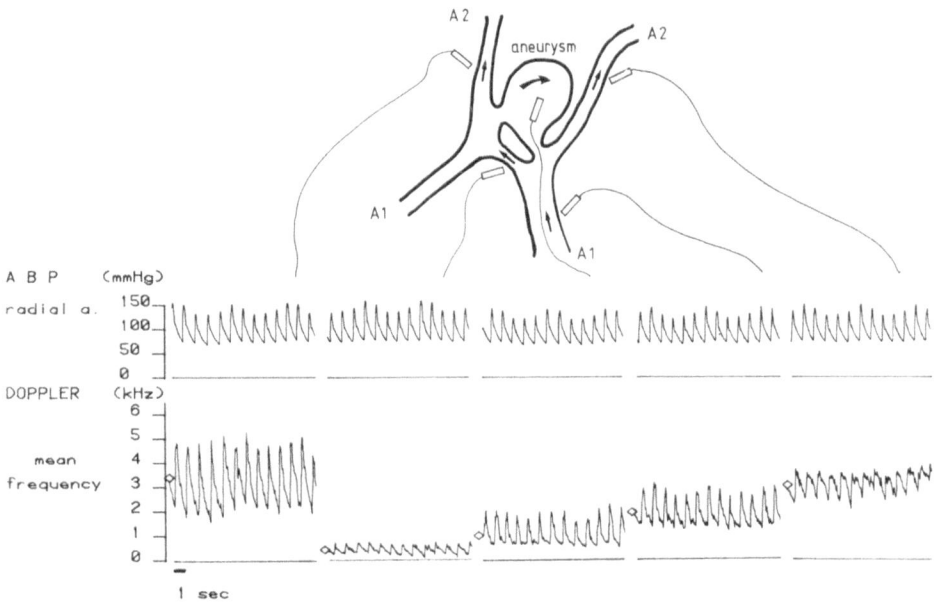

Fig. 48. Aneurysm of the anterior communicating artery (arrow). "Normal" flow pulse waves in the aneurysm and in the anterior system several
weeks after a SAH (to be continued on p. 72)

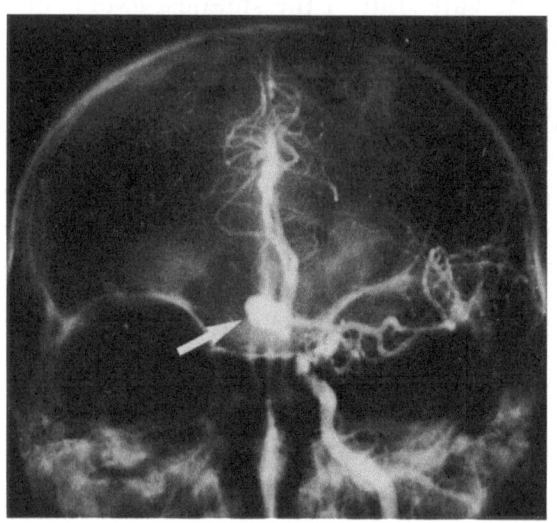

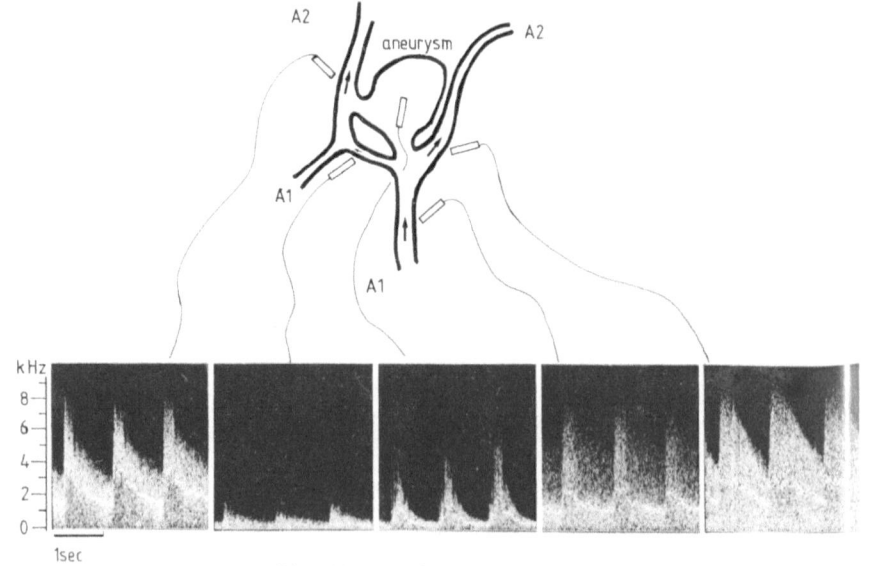

Fig. 48. (continued)

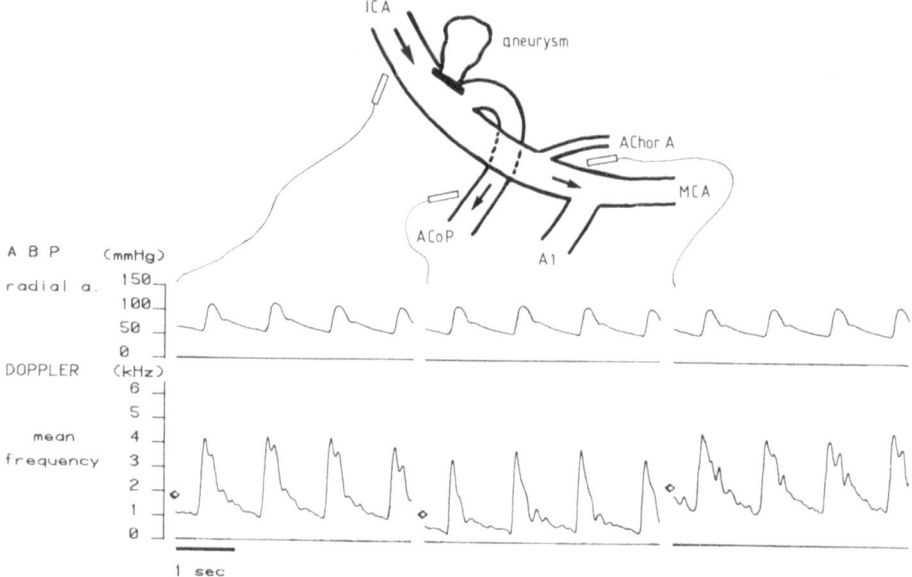

o: time averaged mean

Fig. 49. Aneurysm of the posterior communicating artery. "Normal" flow pulse waves after clipping. Note the relatively high amplitudes accompanying a low diastolic flow as a sign of the increase in resistance in the case of arterial sclerosis

in the internal carotid artery is about the same as that in the main stem of the middle cerebral artery. It is clearly faster in both than in the proximal anterior cerebral artery and in the distal branches of the middle cerebral artery, which have similar velocities.

Table 4. *Mean Doppler frequencies of the most important arteries.* ICA: internal carotid artery, MCA: middle cerebral artery, mca: middle cerebral artery branches, ACA: proximal anterior cerebral artery, aca: distal anterior cerebral artery; SD: standard deviation

| artery | mean frequency (kHz) | | | SD |
	time averaged	systolic	diastolic	
ICA				
normal	3.4	6	1.5	1.1
pathol	3.6	5.4	1.5	1.2

Table 4 (continued)

artery	mean frequency (kHz)			SD
	time averaged	systolic	diastolic	
MCA				
normal	3.3	4.6	1.2	1.0
pathol	4.0	5.4	2.2	1.0
mca				
normal	2.3	4.2	1.0	1.1
pathol	2.6	5.4	1.0	1.1
ACA				
normal	2.8	4.4	0.8	1.1
pathol	3.7	5.8	1.2	1.0
aca				
normal	2.8	4.4	1.0	0.9
pathol	3.5	5.4	1.8	0.9

Spasm and Hyperemia

The flow pulse during acceleration as a result of spasm or of a peripheral reduction in resistance are principally the same. Two waveforms appear regularly: one resembles an upside-down pressure pulse curve with the slowest flow during systole and the fastest flow in diastole (systolic deceleration) (Fig. 50); the other is an irregular waveform with slight amplitude modulation which acoustically resembles a hissing noise (Figs. 51 and 59). The systolic deceleration seems to signal the greater lumen reduction, as is shown by the changeover to the irregular wave after the vessel has been widened with papaverine (Figs. 50, 51 and 54).

The outer diameter is often normal during vasospasms after subarachnoid hemorrhage. One can assess the size of the inner lumen in these cases by employing the automatic gate shift, if possible in comparison with surrounding vessels (Fig. 47). It is easy to distinguish between these cases and general acceleration as a result of hyperemia after recent subarachnoid hemorrhage because in the former, pathological flow pulse waveforms occur everywhere (Figs. 52 and 53).

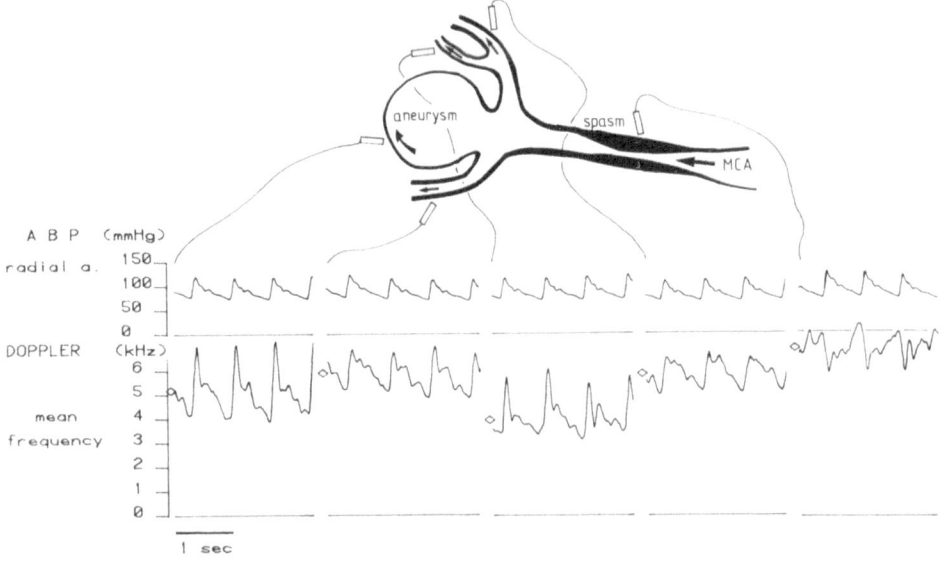

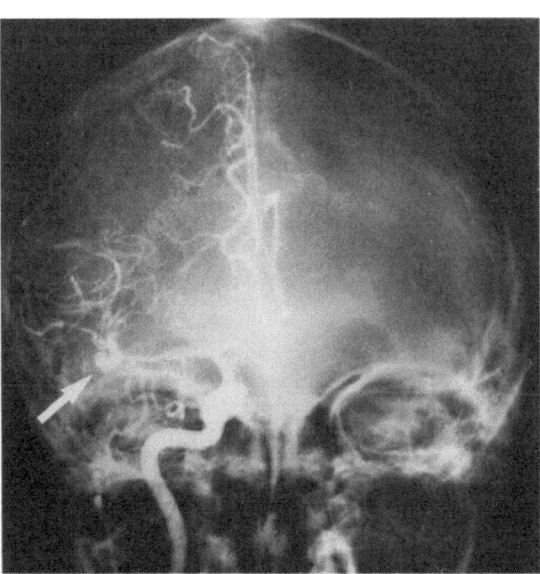

Fig. 50. Aneurysm at the bifurcation of the middle cerebral artery prior to clipping. Note that the flow is on the whole slower in the aneurysm with greater amplitude modulation in comparison to the other vessels. Also note the pathological pulse waveforms with systolic deceleration in the area of a spasm at the main stem of the MCA. (Arrow: aneurysm)

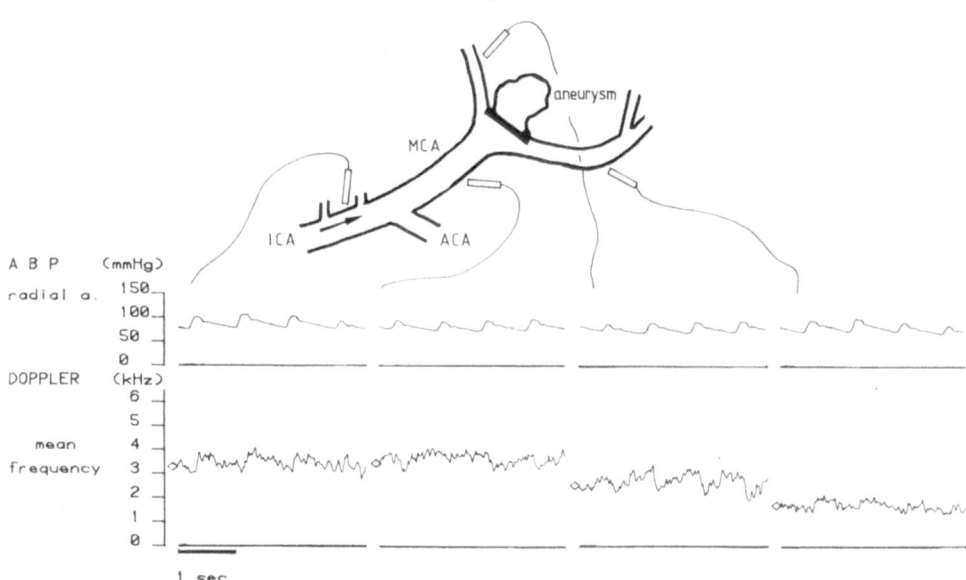

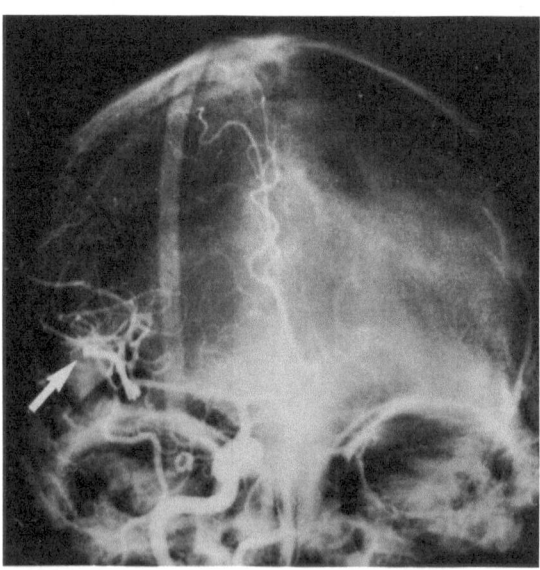

Fig. 51. Aneurysm at the bifurcation of the middle cerebral artery after clipping. Note the changeover of the pulse wave with systolic deceleration to an irregular waveform as a possible sign of a vessel widening caused by dissection and papaverine. (Arrow: clip)

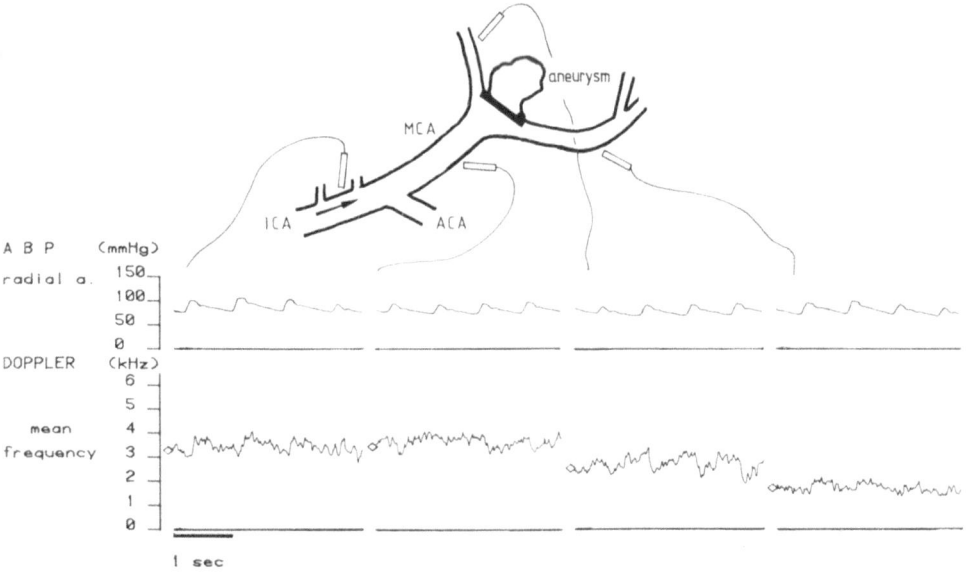

Fig. 52. Aneurysm at the bifurcation of the MCA after clipping. Note the high, unmodulated flow in all the sections as a sign of reduction of resistance (hyperemia) following recent subarachnoid hemorrhage

In accordance with the basic pathomechanism, cross-sectional widening with a deceleration of the flow velocity can be effected with topical papaverine or nimodipine only in spasms that have been mechanically triggered off and that had occurred by bleeding a longer period of time before (Fig. 54). No change can be registered for spasms after SAH dating back 1—2 weeks with normal external vessel caliber.

Early Operation

A high flow with little modulation can be expected in about 75 % of the patients who are operated on within 72 hours after a subarachnoid hemorrhage. In the majority of cases (71 %), this is a result of a reduction of resistance (Figs. 52 and 53). Stenosis is the cause only in the few cases when other preceding hemorrhages are known. A comparable hyperemic reaction can also be achieved with temporary clips (Fig. 55).

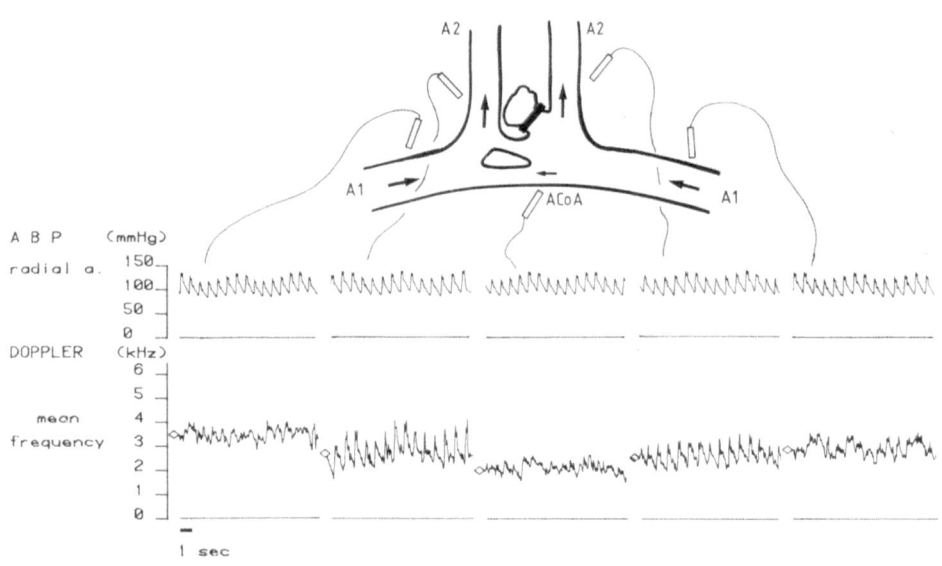

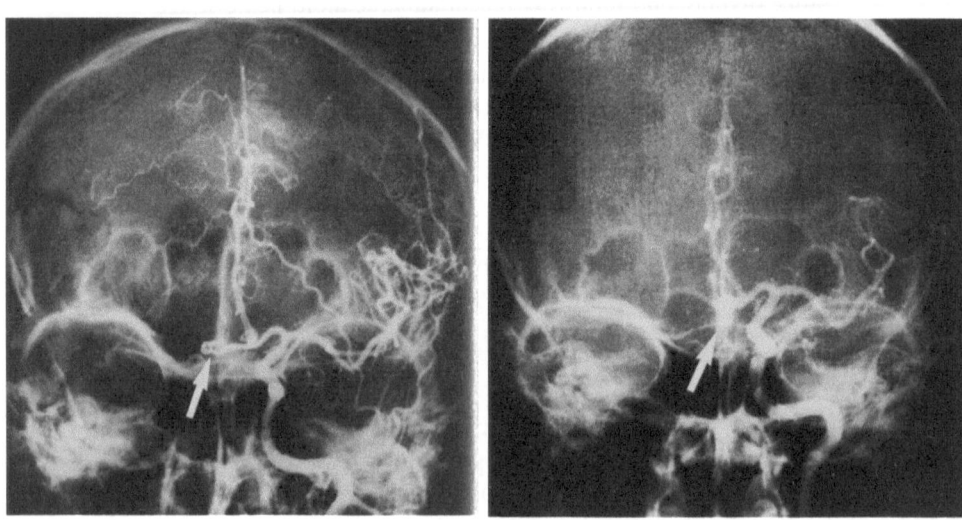

Fig. 53. Anterior communicating artery aneurysm 36 hours after SAH. Note the high unmodulated flow patterns as a sign of hyperemia. Left: immediately before operation (Arrow: aneurysm). Right: immediately after operation (Arrow: clip). Note the relatively wide vessels without vasospasm

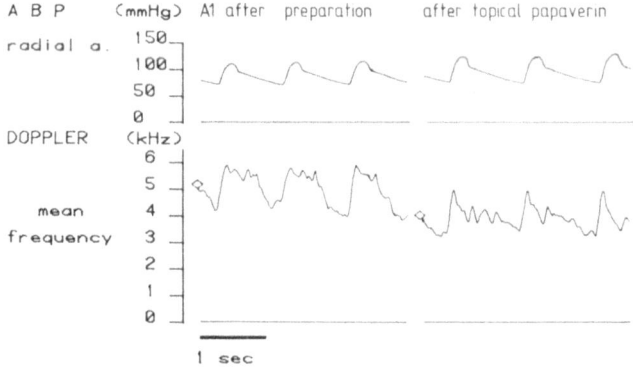

Fig. 54. Vasospasm of the A 1 portion of the anterior cerebral artery with a high flow velocity and irregular flow patterns, which change into a still accelerated but regular pulse curve after topical application of a vaso-dilator

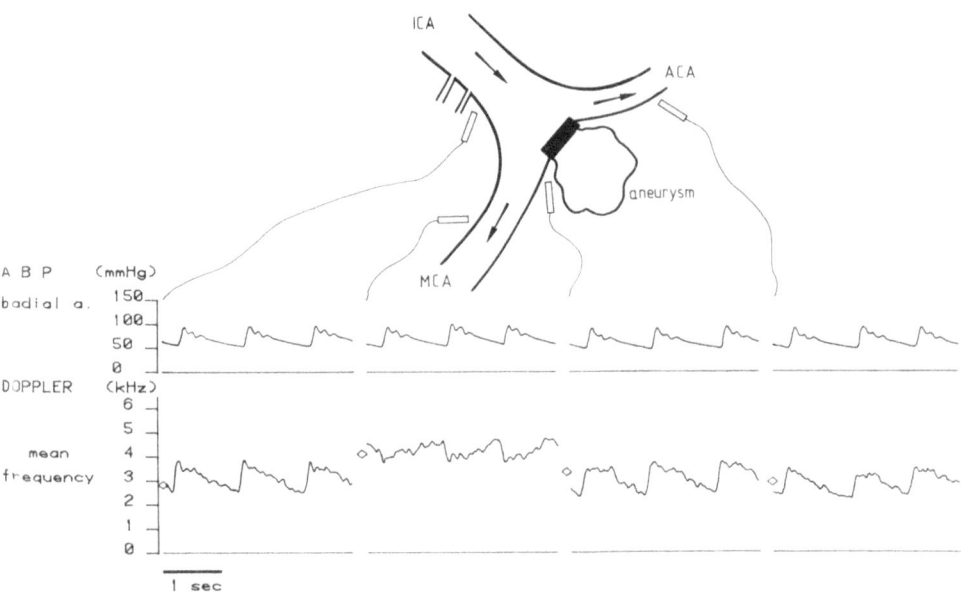

Fig. 55. Doppler control after clipping of a carotid bifurcation aneurysm. Normal flow patterns in the internal carotid artery and anterior cerebral artery; flow acceleration with pathological flow patterns in the middle cerebral artery as a sign of hyperemia after temporary clipping

Artificial Hypotension

In effective pressure reduction (mean pressure between 35 and 60 mm Hg) amplitude modulation is greater at first, the diastolic flow is less, and respiratory modulation is more pronounced. After pressure reduction has been discontinued, a high unmodulated flow due to longer lasting resistance decrease sets in until normalization takes place minutes later (Fig. 56).

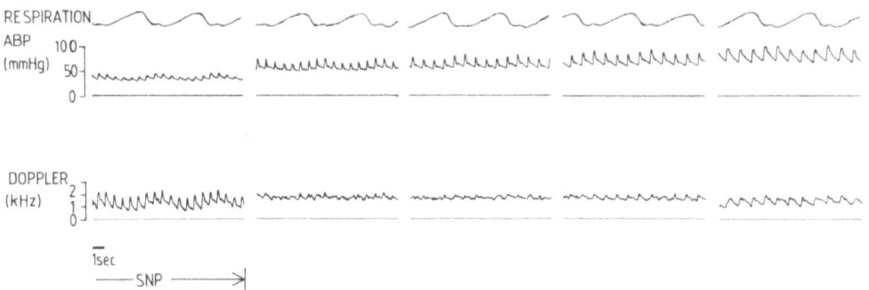

Fig. 56. Pulse waveform change during and after sodium nitroprusside: under vasodilatation and hypotonia flow has a high amplitude with less diastolic flow and with respiratory modulation; hyperemia accompanying continuing SNP effect and rising blood pressure; normalization of pulse and blood pressure as SNP effect ceases

Aneurysm

Intra-aneurysmal flow is surprisingly regular and not turbulent (Figs. 47, 48, 50, and 57). The pulse amplitudes as a rule are higher and more regular than in the supplying vessel; however, the mean Doppler frequencies are lower. Extremely fast (up to 4.2 kHz) and extremely slow (0.2 kHz) intra-aneurysmal Doppler frequencies, which are partly dependent on the size of the neck, are possible.

Studies on 53 cases show that in about 10 %, Doppler sonography yields further information above and beyond the visual impression: in 4 cases complete clipping could be assured despite uncertainties caused by poor visibility of the clipping; in one case the aneurysm was still open, despite a

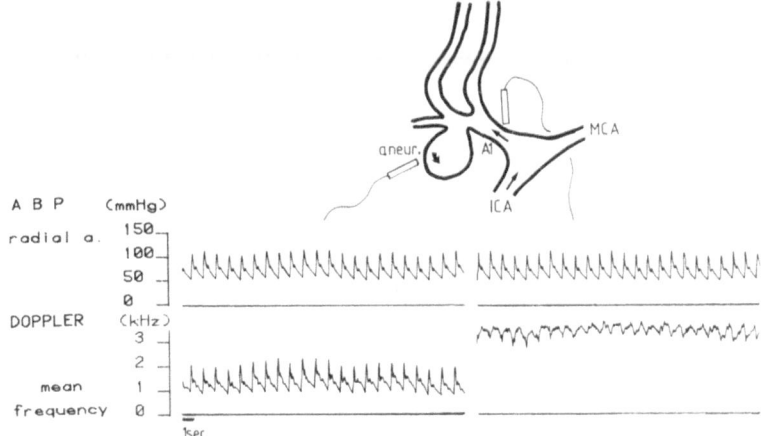

Fig. 57. Anterior communicating artery aneurysm. Note the high velocity and partially irregular flow patterns in the parent anterior cerebral artery and the normal flow pulse curve in the aneurysm

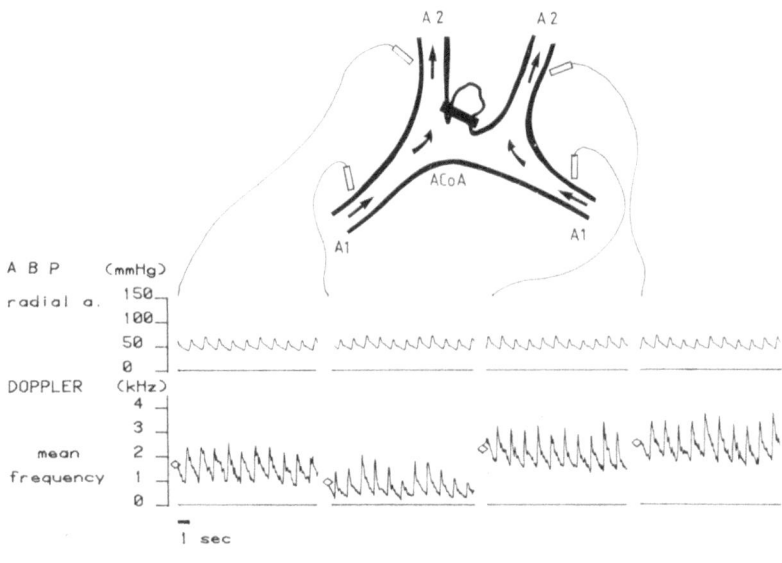

o: time averaged mean

Fig. 58. Anterior communicating artery aneurysm. Normal flow patterns and frequencies in the parent arteries. Variations of Doppler findings in the sections of the anterior system are in the usual range of about 1 kHz

seemingly well-situated clip. In such cases Doppler sonography saves having to use test puncturing, which sometimes ends with surprises.

Parent and Neighboring Vessels

Approximately 90 % of the Doppler sonographic measurements (48 out of 53) correspond to the impression gained under the operation microscope (Figs. 47, 49, 51, 52, 53, and 58). Exceptions to this are the tunnel clips, where the patency can only be evaluated by Doppler sonography (Fig. 59).

In about 10 % of the parent and neighboring vessels, there can be severe lumen reduction or an occlusion, despite outwardly inconspicuous conditions including a well-sitting clip and clear pulsations. Large aneurysms with plaques are predestined for this (Fig. 60).

Anastomoses following aneurysm resections can also be occluded, despite seemingly normal anastomotic conditions and good pulsations. Once detected by Doppler sonography, they can be corrected immediately (Fig. 61).

The absence of flow is an unmistakable sign of a total occlusion. Severe stenoses are indicated by signs of increase in resistance proximal to the clip and slow, low-amplitude flow distal to the clip (Fig. 60). A comparison with the measurements taken before clipping and on neighboring vessels can confirm the flow reduction findings. Examinations on the site of the clip itself for the purpose of finding local acceleration are usually impossible due to the cramped conditions.

Control Angiography

The Doppler method is very reliable, as shown by 45 comparisons with postoperative angiographies performed immediately after surgery (Figs. 51, 53 and 59). The aneurysm exclusion assumed by Doppler sonography and the patency of the vessel correlated in every case. With Doppler sonography vessels with pronounced angiospasms could al-

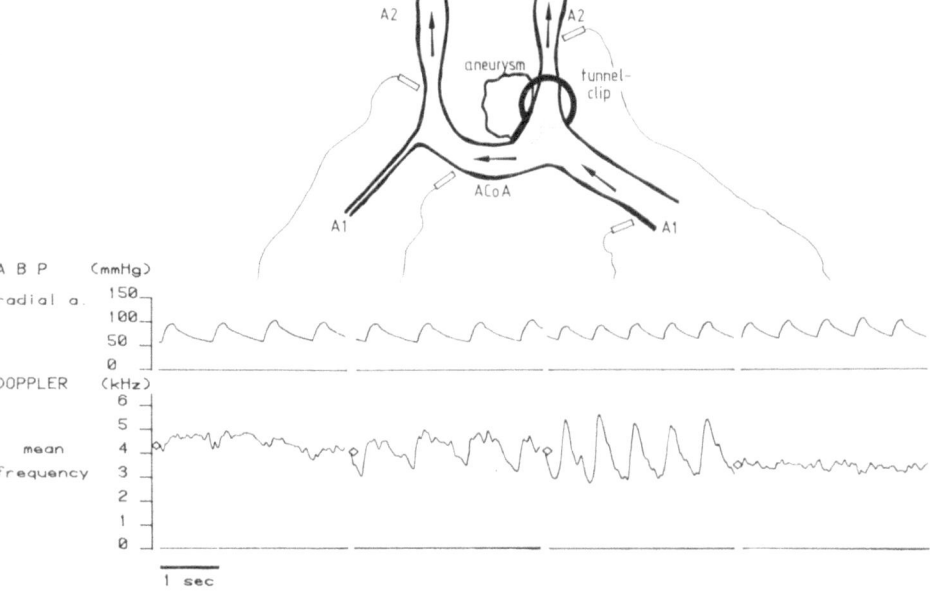

ABP (mmHg)
radial a. 150
100
50
0

DOPPLER (kHz)
6
5
mean 4
frequency 3
2
1
0

1 sec

o: time averaged mean

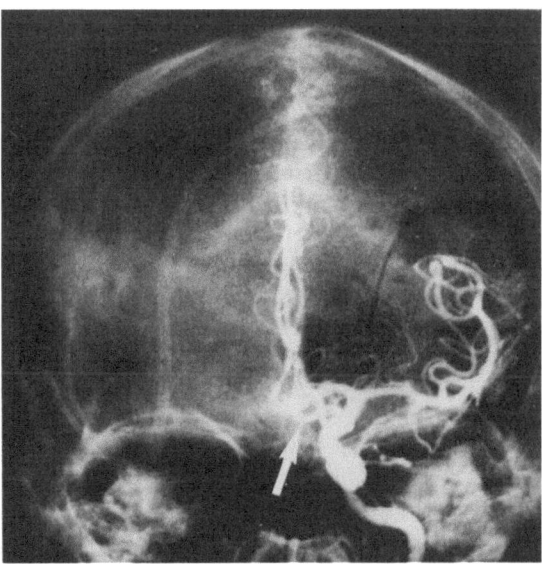

Fig. 59. Anterior communicating artery aneurysm directed dorsally. Exclusion with a tunnel clip. Because of invisible portions the patency of the vessel must be proved by Doppler sonography. Note the flow acceleration with irregularities in the spastic parts of both A2 segments. (Arrow: tunnel clip)

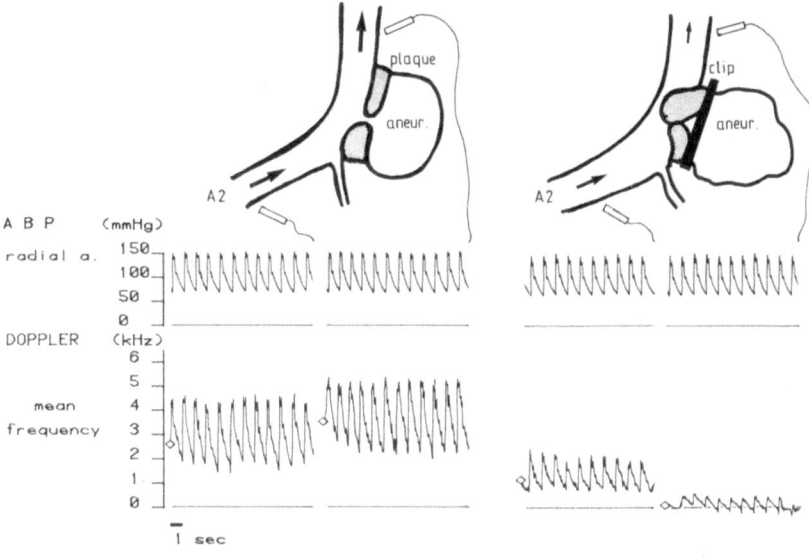

Fig. 60. Distal anterior cerebral artery aneurysm with plaques. Note the
radical reduction in flow velocity after the clip is placed

ready be detected intraoperatively (Fig. 59). Some of the vessels with marked acceleration in flow had a normal caliber, in cases when there had been recent subarachnoid hemorrhages or older dissoluble spasms. More moderate spasms were sometimes preceded by normal Doppler findings. There was no case of normal Doppler findings when the angiography established severe spasms.

Discussion

In contrast to surface animal-experimental and cortical recordings, in carrying out measurement on the base of the brain it is not always possible to achieve an ideal angular adjustment between the probe and the vessel. The essential information is obtained therefore by evaluating the Doppler frequencies before and after clipping recorded at the same place and, as far as possible, at the same angle, and by inter-

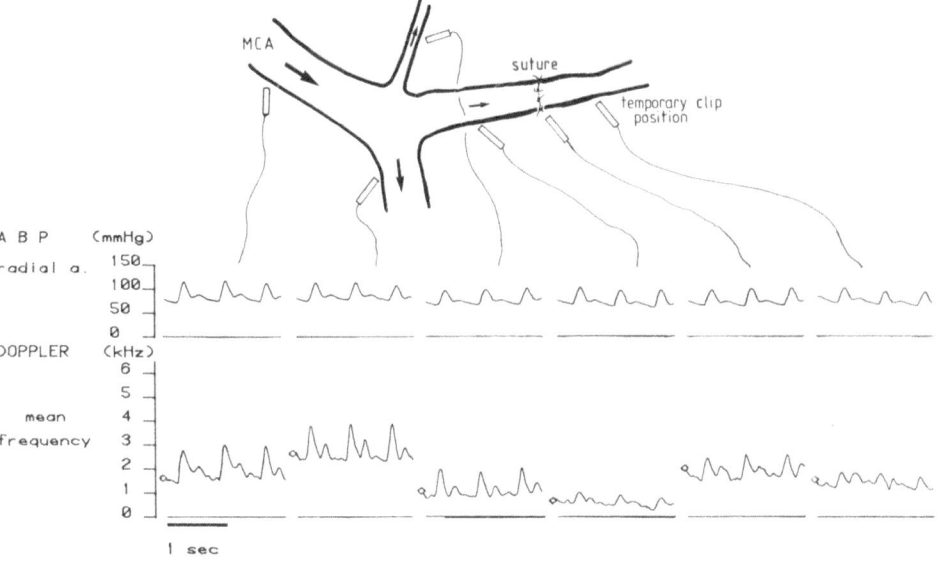

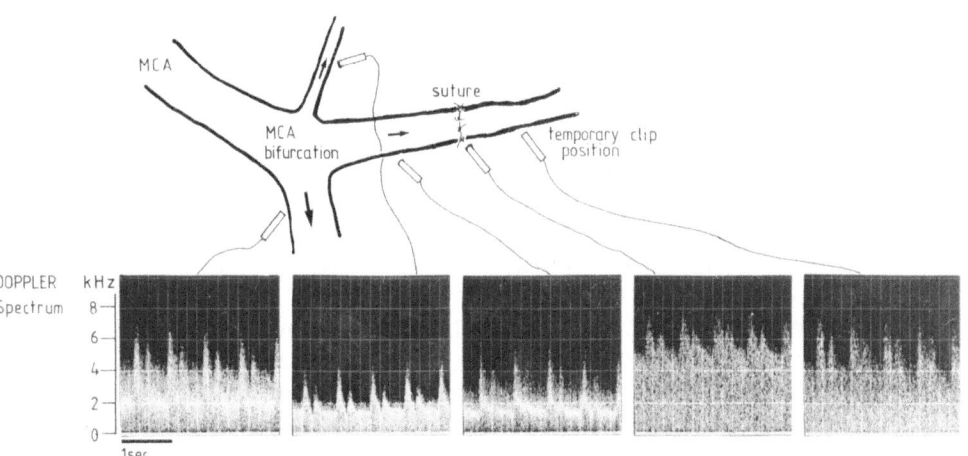

Fig. 61. Middle cerebral artery aneurysm treated by resection and end-to-end suture. Irregularities, acceleration and proximal flow velocity reduction as a sign of a patent but hemodynamically imperfect anastomosis

preting the pulse waveforms, which are relatively independent of the angles.

Recognizing and judging lumen reduction on the basis of local acceleration, as has been described by Nornes et al.[135], poses problems. It is often impossible to carry out the necessary comparison measurement proximal and distal to the tight clip because the clip interferes with the measurement. In cases of spasm, the narrowing is often so extended that control measurement for quantification cannot be taken in the portion of normal caliber.

In spite of these restrictions, the Doppler method makes it possible to control and, if necessary, correct instantly with a high degree of reliability the operative measures in the visible and manipulatable area. This can be done at the latest when these measures become hemodynamically effective, if not before.

Normal Doppler sonographic findings in the circle of Willis were not known until now. The pulse waveform corresponds essentially to that of the cervical carotid artery, but has a broader spectrum, which is common among smaller vessels[51]. In spite of very different pressures, caliber, vessel condition, and recording conditions, the mean Doppler frequencies in the internal carotid artery, the anterior cerebral artery, and the middle cerebral artery remain relatively constant. In clinical practice, to arrive at an approximate value in normal pulse waves it has proved workable to take the mean Doppler frequency, measured in kHz, as corresponding to the diameter of the vessel in millimeters. This means that for typical diameters[201], mean Doppler frequencies with the 20 MHz device for the internal carotid artery are usually about 3.3 kHz, for the middle cerebral artery about 2.3 kHz, and for the anterior cerebral artery around 1.8 kHz.

Information regarding Doppler findings in spasms has only been provided by Nornes et al.[135]. However, high velocities are not found to the extent which Nornes observed.

The inaccuracies associated with determining the cross-section of the vessel with the automatic gate shift and those with pre- and postoperative angiography limit the possibility of determining the degree of spasm: according to studies done so far, the pulse waveforms with systolic deceleration correspond to lumen reductions of 60—80 %, while flow irregularities correspond to lower reductions. There are no examples for lumen area reduction of more than 80 %. A quantification using velocity comparisons in front of and behind the stenosis is hardly practicable due to the limited recording conditions (see above).

The previously unknown high flow velocities with pathological flow pulse waveforms of wide vessels associated with a recent subarachnoid hemorrhage can be interpreted as a peripheral reduction in resistance (hyperemia). This correlates with the findings of Fox et al.[60] and Weir et al.[192], who observed wide and slack vessels in angiograms carried out after recent subarachnoid hemorrhages.

The findings in cases of artificial hypotension with sodium nitroprusside show, apart from the typical waveform change after resistance reduction and simultaneously occurring low pressure, the consequences, of sustained vasodilation in cases of normal and also of high blood pressure after the vasodilator has been discontinued. Cerebral circulation increases, as is known from measurements taken with radioisotopes or electroflowmeters[132, 145].

Since there have been no recordings made while hypotension is being induced, the feasible assessment of the autoregulatory lower limit as Nornes et al.[132] established it with electromagnetic measurements, is not possible.

In contrast to common opinion derived up till now from angiographic and experimental studies[57, 71], Doppler sonographic examinations show a regular and not a turbulent flow. With pulsed high frequency Doppler sonography with small gates, tiny partial volumina can be measured in regular flow streams. Accordingly, when larger gates are used, regular flow is found only in a part of the aneurysms[135].

The higher intra-aneurysmal flow velocities which Nornes et al.[135] described are seldom observed in our patients. Although the aneurysm can be distinguished from normal cerebral arteries by Doppler sonography, personal experience demonstrates that it is not necessary to utilize the localizing and identifying possibilities of Doppler sonography which Nornes et al.[135] have recommended for the operation.

Eight per cent of the vessels contributing to the aneurysms cannot be recorded with Doppler sonography. The reason for this is the size of the probe, which is still somewhat too large. However, it should be possible to reduce the size of the probe, as Freed et al.[63] have described.

The Doppler sonographic method is so reliable that post-operative angiography for patency and clipping control is indicated only if the vessels cannot be recorded or if a residual aneurysm neck between the clip and the vessel cannot be ruled out by visual examination.

Conclusions

In over 90 % of the vessels that can be recorded, microvascular Doppler sonography is an atraumatic and reliable method of testing the clipping of the aneurysm, the patency of the parent artery and of the vessel anastomoses. Hindrances to the vascular system are discovered at the latest when they become hemodynamically effective. Postoperative angiography for patency and clipping control is only necessary in the exceptional case.

Flow acceleration and pathological flow pulse waves can be expected in about 75 % of the patients. This is caused by spasms, which often cannot be recognized externally, or by peripheral resistance reductions following recent subarachnoid hemorrhage.

References

1. Acland, R. D.: Signs of patency in small vessel anastomosis. Surgery 72, 744—748 (1972).
2. Acland R. D., Trachtenberg, L.: The histopathology of small arteries following experimental microvascular anastomosis. Plast. Reconstr. Surg. 60, 868—875 (1977).
3. Albanese, V., Tomasello, F., Cioffi, F. A.: Small arterial anastomoses: Experimental model applicable to microneurosurgical practice. J. Neurosurg. Sci. 19, 40—44 (1975).
4. Anliker, M., Casty, M., Friedli, P., et al.: Noninvasive measurement of blood flow. In: Hwang, N. H. C. (ed.): Cardiovascular Flow Dynamics. University Park Press, 1976.
5. Anliker, M.: Diagnostic analysis of arterial flow pulses in man. In: Baan, J., Nordergraaf, A., Raines, J. (eds.): Cardiovascular System Dynamics, pp. 113—123. Cambridge: MIT Press, 1978.
6. Ausman, J. I., Diaz, F. G.: Correlation of noninvasive Doppler and angiographic evaluation of extra-intracranial anastomoses. In: Peerless, S. J., McCormick, C. W. (eds.): Microsurgery for Cerebral Ischemia, pp. 125—127. Berlin – Heidelberg – New York: Springer, 1980.
7. Austin, G. M., Zimmerman, D.: Prediction of relative flow deficit and EC-IC effectiveness by computer model of circle of Willis. J. Cerebral Blood Flow and Metabolism 1, suppl. 1, 497 (1981).
8. Azuma, T., Fukushima, T.: Flow patterns in stenotic blood vessel models. Biorheology 13, 337—355 (1976).
9. Bakay, L., Sweet, W. H.: Cervical and intracranial intraarterial pressure with and without vascular occlusion. Surg. Gynec. Obstet. 95, 67—75 (1952).
10. Bakay, L., Sweet, W. H.: Intraarterial pressures in the neck and brain. Late changes after carotid closure. J. Neurosurg. 10, 353—359 (1953).
11. Baker, D. W.: Pulsed ultrasonic Doppler-flow sensing. I. E. E. E. Transactions on Sonics and Ultrasonics 17, 170—185 (1970).
12. Baker, D. W.: Applications of pulsed Doppler techniques. Radiologic Clinics of North America 18, 79—103 (1980).
13. Baker, D. W., Steggal, H. F., Schlegel, W. A.: A sonic transcutaneous blood flowmeter: Proc. 17th Conf. Engng. Med. Biol. 76, (1964).
14. Baldes, E. J., Farral, W. R., Haugen, M. C.: A forum on an ultrasonic

method for measuring the velocity in blood. In: Kelly, E. (ed.): Ultrasound in Biology and Medicine, p. 165. Washington: Amer. Inst. Biol. Sc., 1957.

15. Banis, J. C., Schwartz, K. S., Acland, R. D.: Electromagnetic flowmetry — an experimental method for continuous blood flow measurement using a new island flap model. Plast. Reconstr. Surg. *66*, 534—544 (1980).

16. Beasley, M. G., Blau, J. N., Gosling, R. G.: Changes in internal carotid artery flow velocities with cerebral vasodilatation and constriction. Stroke *10*, 331—335 (1979).

17. van Beek, A. L., Link, W. J., Bennett, J. E.: Ultrasound evaluation of microanastomosis. Arch. Surg. *110*, 945—949 (1975).

18. Bellman, S., Koevamees, A., Rietz, K.-A.: Reconstruction of small arteries: Androsov's and Nakayama's apparatuses and microangiography. In: Donaghy, R. M. P., Yaşargil, M. G. (eds.): Microvascular Surgery, pp. 67—74. Stuttgart: G. Thieme, 1967.

19. Berguer, R., Hwang, N. H. C.: Critical arterial stenosis: a theoretical and experimental solution. Ann. Surg. *180*, 39—50 (1974).

20. Blair, W. F., Greene, E. R., Omer, G. E.: A method for the calculation of blood flow in human digital arteries. J. Hand. Surg. *6*, 90—96 (1981).

21. Blair, W. F., Greene, E. R., Eldridge, M., *et al.*: Hemodynamics after microsurgical anastomosis: the effects of topical lidocaine. J. Microsurg. *2*, 157—164 (1981).

22. Bradley, E. L., Saceri, O.: The velocity of ultrasound in human blood under varying physiologic parameters. J. Surg. Res. *12*, 290—297 (1972).

23. Brambilla, G., Paoletti, P., Rodriguez y Baena, R.: Extracranial-intracranial arterial bypass in the treatment of inoperable giant aneurysms of the internal carotid artery. Acta Neurochir. (Wien) *60*, 63—69 (1982).

24. Brandestini, A.: Topoflow — a digital full range Doppler velocity meter. I. E. E. E. Transactions on Sonics and Ultrasonics. SU *25*, 287—293 (1978).

25. Brawley, B. W.: Determination of superior sagittal sinus patency with an ultrasonic doppler flow detector in parasagittal meningioma. J. Neurosurg. *30*, 315—316 (1969).

26. Buedingen, H. J., von Reutern, G.-M., Freund, H.-J.: Dopplersonographie der extrakraniellen Hirnarterien. Stuttgart - New York: G. Thieme, 1982.

27. Buedingen, H. J., von Reutern, G.-M.: Atraumatische Vorfelddiagnostik des Hirntodes mit der Doppler-Sonographie. Dtsch. med. Wschr. *104*, 1347—1351 (1979).

28. Buedingen, H. J., Gilsbach, J., von Reutern, G.-M.: Dopplersonographische Therapie- und Verlaufskontrolle einer katheteroccludierten Cavernosusfistel. Arch. Psychiat. Nervenkr. *226*, 19—27 (1978).

29. Busse, R., Pasch, Th.: Arterielle Strompulsformen — Entstehung und transkutane Registrierung. In: Kriessmann, A., Bollinger, A. (eds.): Ultraschall-Doppler-Diagnostik in der Angiologie. Stuttgart: G. Thieme, 1977.

30. Byar, D., Fiddian, R. V., Quereau, M., et al.: The fallacy of applying the Poiseuille equation to segmental arterial stenosis. Am. Heart J. 70, 216—224 (1963).

31. Cannon, J. A., Lobpreis, E. L., Herrold, G., et al.: Experience with a new electromagnetic flowmeter for use in blood-flow determinations in surgery. Ann. Surg. 152, 635—646 (1960).

32. Carter, L. P., White, W. L., Atkinson, D. R.: Regional cortical blood flow at craniotomy. Neurosurgery 2, 223—229 (1978).

33. Carter, L. P., Erspamer, R. B. S., White, W. L., et al.: Cortical blood flow during craniotomy for aneurysm. Surg. Neurol. 17, 204—208 (1982).

34. Carter, L. P., Erspamer, R. J.: Regional cortical blood flow during cerebrovascular surgery. In: Peerless, S. J., McCormick, C. W. (eds.): Microsurgery for Cerebral Ischemia, pp. 40—45. Berlin – Heidelberg – New York: Springer, 1980.

35. Cathignol, P., Chapelon, J. Y., Fourcade, C.: Vélocimètre Doppler à l'usage des petits vaisseaux, le Microflo. Biosigma (Paris), pp. 426—429, 1978.

36. Cathignol, D., Fourcade, C.: Improvement of Pulsed Doppler Flowmeter for Use in Microvascular Diagnosis. ICEU New Delhi A 13, 18—20 (1980).

37. Cathignol, D., Chapelon, J. Y., Mestas, J. L., et al.: Description et application d'un vélocimètre ultrasonore Doppler pour les petits vaisseaux. Med. & Biol. Eng. & Comput 21, 358—364 (1983).

38. Chang, J. L., Albin, M. S., Bunegin, L. B. S., et al.: Analysis and comparison of venous air embolism detection methods. Neurosurgery 7, 135—141 (1980).

39. Chater, N.: Surgical results and measurments of intraoperative flow in microsurgical anastomoses. In: Austin, G. M., Thomas, C. C. (eds.): Microneurosurgical Anastomoses for Cerebral Ischemia, pp. 295—304. Springfield, Ill.: Ch. C Thomas, 1976.

40. Choi, H. K., Stowe, N., Novick, A.: Comparison of end-to-end with telescoped arterial anastomoses in renal transplantation in rats. J. Microsurg. 3, 85—88 (1981).

41. Collice, M., Scialfa, G., Valsecchi, F., et al.: Cortical artery pressure: preoperative and postoperative arteriographic finding in patients with internal carotid artery occlusion. In: Peerless, S. J., McCormick, C. W. (eds.): Microsurgery for Cerebral Ischemia, pp. 138—141. Berlin – Heidelberg – New York: Springer, 1980.

42. Collice, M., Fornari, M., Porta, M.: End-to-side anastomosis between carotid arteries and serial angiographic controls in rats. In: Schmiedek, P. (ed.): Microsurgery for Stroke, pp. 159—162. Berlin – Heidelberg — New York: Springer, 1977.

43. Cook, A. F., Grossman, J. A. I., Herpy, E. S., *et al.*: A method for quantitative analysis of lumen changes in microvascular anastomoses. J. Microsurg. *3*, 54—55 (1981).
44. Corwin, T. R., Bingham, H. G.: The Doppler and its use in axial flaps. Am. J. Surg. *131*, 660—663 (1976).
45. Coulter, N. A., Pappenheimer, J. R.: Development of turbulence in flowing blood. Amer. J. Physiol. *159*, 401 (1949).
46. Crowell, R. M.: Electromagnetic flow studies of superficial temporal artery to middle cerebral branch artery bypass graft. In: Austin, G. M. (ed.): Microsurgical Anastomoses for Cerebral Ischemia, pp. 116—124. Springfield, Ill.: Ch. C Thomas, 1976.
47. Daniel, R. D., Terzis, J. K. (eds.): Reconstructive Microsurgery, pp. 83—85. Boston: Little, Brown & Co, 1977.
48. Diaz, F. G., Ausman, J. I., Pearce, J. E.: Ischemic complications after combined internal carotid artery occlusion and extracranial-intracranial anastomosis. Neurosurgery *10*, 563—570 (1982).
49. Dieckhoff, D., Kanzow, E.: Über die Lokalisation des Strömungswiderstandes im Hirnkreislauf. Pfluegers Arch. *310*, 75—85 (1969).
50. Diener, H. C., Voigt, K., Dichgans, J.: Diagnosis of intracranial malformations by Doppler sonography. Neurochirurgia *24*, 185—191 (1981).
51. van Dongen, M. E. H., van Steenhoven, A. A.: Some fluid dynamical aspects of arterial flow. In: Reneman, R. S., Hoeks, A. P. G. (eds.): Doppler Ultrasound in the Diagnosis of Cerebrovascular Disease, pp. 29—58. Chichester – New York – Brisbane – Toronto – Singapore: Research Studies Press, 1982.
52. Doppler, C.: Ueber das farbige Licht der Doppelsterne und einiger anderer Gestirne des Himmels. Abh. Kgl. Boehm. Ges. d. Wissensch. (Prag) 1842, pp. 465—482.
53. Drake, C. G., Vanderlinden, R. G.: The late consequences of incomplete surgical treatment of cerebral aneurysms. J. Neurosurg. *27*, 226—238 (1967).
54. Eldridge, M. W., Greene, E. R., Berman, W. R., *et al.*: Ultrasonic pulsed Doppler characterization of the human neonatal peripheral circulation. Biomed. Sci. Instrum. *15*, 77—90 (1979).
55. Feindel, W., Yamamoto, Y. L., Hodge, C. P.: Red cerebral veins and the cerebral steal syndrome. Evidence from fluorescein angiography and microregional blood flow by radioisotopes during excision of an angioma. J. Neurosurg. *35*, 167—179 (1971).
56. Feindel, W., Yamamoto, Y. L., Hodge, C. P.: The cerebral microcirculation in man: analysis by radioisotope microregional flow measurement and fluorescein angiography, pp. 225—246. In: Tindall, G. T., Wilkins, R. H., Keener, E. B. (eds.): Clinical Neurosurgery, Vol. 18. Baltimore: Williams and Wilkins, 1971.
57. Ferguson, G. G.: Turbulence in human intracranial saccular aneurysms. J. Neurosurg. *33*, 485—487 (1970).
58. Ferguson, G. G.: Direct measurement of mean and pulsatile blood

pressure at operation in human intracranial saccular aneurysms. J. Neurosurg. *36*, 560—563 (1972).

59. Foroglou, G.: Contribution de l'écho-encéphalographie au diagnostic de la mort cérébrale. Schweiz. med. Wschr. *104*, 1291—1294 (1974).

60. Fox, J. L., Ko, L.: Cerebral vasospasm: a clinical observation. Surg. Neurol. *10*, 269—275 (1978).

61. Franklin, D. L., Schlegel, W. A., Rushmer, R. F.: Blood flow measured by Doppler frequency shift of back scattered ultrasound. Science *132*, 564—565 (1961).

62. Freed, D., Hartley, C. J., Christman, K. D., *et al.*: Pulsed Doppler flow estimation in small vessels. Proc. of 31st annual conference on engineering in medicine and biology 1978, p. 190.

63. Freed, D., Hartley, C. J., Christman, K. D., *et al.*: High-frequency pulsed Doppler ultrasound: a new tool for microvascular surgery. J. Microsurg. *1*, 148—153 (1979).

64. Freund, H. J.: Personal communication 1975.

65. Friedrich, H., Haensel-Friedrich, G., Seeger, W.: Intraoperative Dopplersonographie an Hirngefaessen. Neurochirurgia *23*, 89—98 (1980).

66. Fuentes, J. M.: Cortical arterial pressure in extra-intracranial anastomosis. Acta Neurochir. (Wien) Suppl. 28, 272—274 (1979).

67. Fuentes, J. M., Cesari, J. B., Prince, P.: Place du "Doppler" dans le bilan pré et postopératoire des anastomoses extra-intracrâniennes (à propos de 40 cas). Ultrasons *1*, 301—308 (1980).

68. Fukasawa, H.: Hemodynamical studies of cerebral arteries by means of mathematical analysis of arterial casts. Tohoku J. Exptl. Med. *99*, 255—268 (1969).

69. Gelber, B. R., Sundt, T. M.: Treatment of intracavernous and giant carotid aneurysms by combined internal carotid ligation and extra to intracranial bypass. J. Neurosurg. *52*, 1—10 (1980).

70. George, P., Pourcelot, L., Fourcade, C., *et al.*: Effet Doppler et mesure du débit sanguin. C. R. Acad. Sc. Paris *261*, 253—256 (1965).

71. German, W. J., Black, S. P. W.: Intra-aneurysmal hemodynamics: turbulence. Trans. Am. Neurol. Assoc. *79*, 163—165 (1954).

72. Gildenberg, P. L., O'Brien, R. P., Britt, W. J., *et al.*: The efficacy of Doppler monitoring for the detection of venous air embolism. J. Neurosurg. *54*, 75—78 (1981).

73. Gosling, R. G.: General discussion: the usefulness of zero-crossing meters. In: Reneman, R. S. (ed.): Cardiovascular applications of ultrasound, pp. 455—456. Amsterdam – London – New York: North-Holland / American Elsevier, 1974.

74. Gould, K. L., Lipscomb, K., Calvert, C.: Compensatory changes of the distal coronary vascular bed during progressive coronary constriction. Circulation *51*, 1085 (1975).

75. Greene, E. R., Blair, W. F., Hartley, C. J.: Noninvasive pulsed Dopp-

ler velocity measurements and calculated flow in human digital arteries. Biomed. Sci. Instrum. *16*, 93—105 (1980).

76. Haerten, R.: Technische Kenngrößen von Ultraschalldiagnosegeräten und ihre Bestimmung. Ultraschall *1*, 1—11 (1980).

77. Handa, H., Moritake, K., Nagata, J., *et al.*: Intraoperative hemodynamic study by Doppler ultrasonic flowmeter in the extracranial-intracranial arterial bypass. In: Peerless, S. J., McCormick, C. W. (eds.): Microsurgery for Cerebral Ischemia, pp. 99—105. Berlin – Heidelberg – New York: Springer, 1980.

78. Hartley, C. J., Cole, J. S.: An ultrasonic pulsed Doppler system for measuring blood flow in small vessels. J. Appl. Physiol. *37*, 626—629 (1974).

79. Hayhurst, J. W., O'Brien, B.: An experimental study of microvascular technique, patency rates, and related factors. Brit. J. Plast. Surg. *28*, 128 (1975).

80. Hitchon, P. W., Kassell, N. F., McDonnell, D. E.: The Doppler ultrasonic flowmeter as an adjunct to operative management of cerebral arteriovenous malformations. Surg. Neurol. *11*, 345—347 (1979).

81. Hoeks, A. P. G., Reneman, R. S., Peronneau, P. A.: A multi-gate pulsed Doppler system with serial data processing. I. E. E. E. Transactions on Sonics and Ultrasonics *28*, 242—247 (1981).

82. Hopkins, L. N., Grand, W.: Extracranial-intracranial arterial bypass in the treatment of aneurysms of the carotid and middle cerebral arteries. Neurosurgery *5*, 21—31 (1979).

83. Hunt, W. E., Hess, R. M.: Surgical risk as related to time of intervention in the repair of intracranial aneurysms. J. Neurosurg. *28*, 14—19 (1968).

84. Ikeda, K.: Cerebral angiography of the rat. J. Neurosurg. *49*, 319—321 (1978).

85. Ito, Z., Hen, R., Nakajima, K., *et al.*: Selection of completed stroke patients for STA-MCA anastomosis based on measurements of somatosensory evoked potential and CBF dynamics. In: Peerless, S. J., McCormick, C. W. (eds.): Microsurgery for Cerebral Ischemia, pp. 177—184. Berlin – Heidelberg – New York: Springer, 1980.

86. Jacobs, G. B., Byer, A., Hubbard, J. H., *et al.*: Doppler ultrasonic mapping of the superficial temporal artery. In: Dietz, H., Metzel, E., Langmaid, C. (eds.): Neurological Surgery, Supplement to Neurochirurgia, p. 384. Stuttgart – New York: G. Thieme, 1981.

87. Jorgensen, J. E., Campau, D. J., Baker, D. W.: Physical characteristic and mathematical modelling of pulse ultrasonic flowmeter. Med. Biol. Engng. *12*, 404—429 (1973).

88. Kalmus, H. P.: Electronic flowmeter system. Rev. Sci. Instr. *25*, 201 (1954).

89. Kaneko, Z., Shiraishi, J., Omizo, *et al.*: Analysis of ultrasonic blood rheogram by the sound spectrograph. Jap. Circul. J. *34*, 1035—1045 (1970).

90. Kanzow, E., Dieckhoff, D.: On the location of the vascular resis-

tance in the cerebral circulation. In: Brock, M., Fierchi, C., Ingvar, D. H. (eds.): Cerebral Blood Flow, pp. 96—97. Berlin – Heidelberg – New York: Springer, 1969.

91. Kassell, N. F., Boarini, D. J., Adams, H. P., et al.: Overall management of ruptured aneurysms; comparison of early and late operation. Neurosurgery 9, 120—128 (1981).

92. Keller, H. M., Meier, W. E., Anlicker, M.: Noninvasive velocity profile determination in the common carotid artery by means of pulsed Doppler ultrasound: Biomedizinische Technik, Band 21, p. 173. Basel: Medex, 1976.

93. Khalifa, A. M. A., Giddens, D. P.: Analysis of disorder in pulsatile flows with application to poststenotic blood velocity measurement in dogs. J. Biomechanics 11, 129—141 (1978).

94. Khalifa, A. M. A., Giddens, D. P.: Characterisation and evaluation of poststenotic flow disturbances. J. Biomechanics 14, 279—296 (1981).

95. Kodama, N., Suzuki, J.: Bypass surgery in the treatment of aneurysms. Neurosurg. Rev. 5, 87—90 (1982).

96. Krag, C., Holck, S.: The value of the patency test in microvascular anastomosis; correlation between observed patency and size of its intraluminal thrombus: an experimental study in rats. Brit. J. Plast. Surg. 34, 64—66 (1981).

97. Krag, C., Holck, S.: Microvascular anastomoses. A comparison of the end-to-end and the telescope techniques in rats. J. Microsurg. 2, 3—10 (1980).

98. Kreuzer, W., Schenk, W., Jr.: Effects of local vasodilatation on blood flow through arterial stenosis. Eur. Surg. Res. 5, 233—242 (1973).

99. Kriessmann, A., Bollinger, A.: Ultraschall-Doppler-Diagnostik in der Angiologie. Stuttgart: G. Thieme, 1978.

100. Lassen, N. A.: Autoregulation of cerebral blood flow. Circ. Res. 15 (Suppl.), 201—204 (1964).

101. Lassen, N. A., Christensen, M. S.: Physiology of cerebral blood flow. Br. J. Anaesth. 48, 715—734 (1976).

102. Latchaw, R. E., Ausman, J. I., Lee, C.: Superficial temporal-middle cerebral artery bypass. A detailed analysis of multiple pre- and postoperative angiograms in 40 consecutive patients. J. Neurosurg. 51, 455—465 (1979).

103. Lauritzen, C., Bagge, U.: A technical and biomechanical comparison between two types of microvascular anastomoses. Scand. J. Plast. Reconstr. Surg. 13, 417—421 (1979).

104. Lindegaard, K.-F., Grip, A., Bakke, S. J., et al.: Clinical Doppler flow velocity measurements in precerebral artery occlusive disease. Acta Neurochir. (Wien) 56, 129 (1981).

105. Little J. R., Yamamoto, Y. L., Feindel, W., et al.: Superficial temporal artery to middle cerebral artery anastomosis; intraoperative evaluation by fluorescein angiography and xenon-133 clearance. J. Neurosurg. 50, 560—569 (1979).

106. Little, J. R., Yamamoto, Y. L., Feindel, W., et al.: Cerebral blood flow in superficial temporal artery to middle cerebral anastomosis. In: Peerless, S. J., McCormick, C. W. (eds.): Microsurgery for Central Ischemia, pp. 59—60. Berlin - Heidelberg - New York: Springer, 1980.

107. Ljunggren, B., Brandt, L., Kagstroem, E., et al.: Results of early operations for ruptured aneurysms. J. Neurosurg. 54, 473—479 (1981).

108. Logan, S. E.: On the fluid mechanics of human coronary artery stenosis. I. E. E. E. Trans. Biomed. Engng. 22, 327—334 (1975).

109. Loop, J. W., Foltz, E. L.: Applications of angiography during intracranial operation. Acta Radiol. (Diagn.) 5, 363—367 (1966).

110. Luebbers, D. W.: Physiologie der Gehirndurchblutung. In: Gaenshirt, H.: Der Hirnkreislauf, pp. 214—260. Stuttgart: Thieme, 1972.

111. Lunt, M. J.: Accuracy and limitations of the ultrasonic Doppler blood velocimeter and zerocrossing detector. Ultrasound. Med. Biol., Vol. 2, pp. 1—10. Pergamon Press, 1975.

112. McLeod, F. D.: A directional Doppler-flowmeter. Digest. of 7th Intern. Conf. Med. Biol. Engng. (Stockholm) 1967, p. 213.

113. McLeod, F. D.: Multichannel pulse Doppler techniques. In: Reneman, R. S. (ed.): Cardiovascular Applications of Ultrasound, pp. 85—107. Amsterdam — London: North-Holland Publishing Company, New York: American Elsevier Company, 1974.

114. Mann, F. C., Herrick, J. F., Essex, H. E., et al.: The effect on the blood flow of decreasing the lumen of a blood vessel. Surgery 4, 249—252 (1938).

115. Matjasko, M. J., Williams, J. P., Fontanilla, M.: Intraoperative use of Doppler to detect successful obliteration of carotid-cavernous fistulas. Technical note. J. Neurosurg. 43, 634—636 (1975).

116. May, A. G., van de Berg, L., de Weese, J. A., et al.: Critical arterial stenosis. Surgery 54, 250—258 (1963).

117. May, A. G., de Weese, J. A., Rob, C. G.: Hemodynamic effects of arterial stenosis. Surgery 53, 513—524 (1963).

118. Mehdorn, M. H., Chater, N. L, Townsend, J. J., et al.: Giant aneurysms and cerebral ischemia. Surg. Neurol. 13, 49—57 (1980).

119. Meier, W. E., Keller, H.: Der Wert intraoperativer Carotis-Doppler-Sonographie im Hinblick auf Prognose bzw. postoperativen Verlauf. Helv. Chir. Acta 43, 107 (1976).

120. Merory, J., du Boulay, G. H., Marshall, J.: Cerebral blood flow following aneurysmal surgery after subarachnoid hemorrhage. Acta Neurochir. (Wien) 46, 180 (1979).

121. Mesner, J. E., Rushmer, R. F.: Eddy formation and turbulence in flowing liquids. Circ. Res. 12, 455—463 (1963).

122. Meyermann, R., Kletter, G., Koos, W. T.: Morphologic changes after vascular microanastomoses as a function of the technique used. In: Schmieder, P. (ed.): Microsurgery for Stroke, pp. 123—127. Berlin - Heidelberg - New York: Springer, 1977.

123. Mizukami, M., Kin, H., Sakuta, Y., et al.: Cortical arterial pressure in

occlusive cerebrovascular disease and results in bypass surgery. In: Schmiedek, P. (ed.): Microsurgery for Stroke, pp. 233—239. Berlin – Heidelberg – New York: Springer, 1977.

124. Moritake, K., Handa, H., Yonekawa, Y., et al.: Ultrasonic Doppler assessment of hemodynamics in superficial temporal artery-middle cerebral artery anastomosis. Surg. Neurol. 13, 249—257 (1980).

125. Moritake, K., Takebe, Y., Yonekawa, Y.: Ultrasonic Doppler assessment of hemodynamics in superficial temporal artery — middle cerebral artery (STA-MCA) anastomosis. In: Dietz, H., Metzel, E., Langmaid, C.: Neurological Surgery, Supplement to Neurochirurgia, p. 245. Stuttgart: G. Thieme, 1981.

126. Mueller, H. R., Gratzl, O.: Ultrasonic monitoring of superficial temporal artery blood flow in EC/IC bypass operations. In: Meyer, J. S., Lechner, H., Reivich, M. (eds.): Cerebral Vascular Diseases 2, pp. 235—240. Amsterdam – Oxford: Excerpta Medica, 1979.

127. Müller, H. R., Gratzl, O.: Quantitative Funktionsprüfung des ATS/ACM/Bypasses mittels eines neuartigen Ultraschall-Flowmeters. Ultraschall 1, 217—222 (1980).

128. Naumann, C., Jung, W., Schoen, F.: Methoden zur Durchblutungsbestimmung freier Lappentransplantate im Tierexperiment. In: Scheunemann, H., Schmidseder, R. (eds.): Plastische und Wiederherstellungschirurgie bei bösartigen Tumoren, pp. 80—87. Berlin – Heidelberg – New York: Springer, 1982.

129. Nienborgh, L.: Assessing the patency of microvascular anastomoses. Brit. J. Plast. Surg. 32, 151 (1979).

130. Nightingale, G., Fogdestam, I., O'Brien, B. M. C.: Scanning electron microscope study of experimental microvascular anastomoses in the rabbit. Br. J. Plast. Surg. 33, 283—298, 1980.

131. Nornes, H., Wickeby, P.: Cerebral arterial blood flow and aneurysm surgery. Part 1, local arterial flow dynamics. J. Neurosurg. 47, 810—818 (1977).

132. Nornes, H., Knutzen, H. B., Wikeby, P.: Cerebral arterial blood flow and aneurysm surgery. Part 2, Induced hypotension and autoregulatory capacity. J. Neurosurg. 47, 819—827 (1977).

133. Nornes, H., Angelsen, B., Lindegaard, K.-F.: Precerebral arterial blood flow pattern in intracranial hypertension with cerebral blood flow arrest. Acta Neurochir. (Wien) 38, 187—194 (1977).

134. Nornes, H., Grip, A., Wikeby, P.: Intraoperative evaluation of cerebral hemodynamics using directional Doppler technique. Part 1, Arteriovenous malformations. J. Neurosurg. 50, 145—151 (1979).

135. Nornes, H., Grip, A., Wikeby, P.: Intraoperative evaluation of cerebral hemodynamics using directional Doppler technique. Part 2, Saccular aneurysms. J. Neurosurg. 50, 570—577 (1979).

136. Nornes, H., Grip, A.: Hemodynamic aspects of cerebral arteriovenous malformations. J. Neurosurg. 53, 456—464 (1980).

137. Nornes, H., Grip, A.: Studies on hemodynamic effects of the exclu-

sion of cerebral arterio-venous malformations. Acta Neurochir. (Wien) *56*, 134 (1981).

138. Pagnanelli, D. M., Pait, T. G., Rizzoli, H. V., *et al.*: Scanning electron micrographic study of vascular lesions caused by microvascular needles and suture. J. Neurosurg. *53*, 32—36 (1980).

139. Parkinson, D.: Cerebral arteriovenous aneurysms; surgical management. Can. J. Surg. *1*, 313—325 (1958).

140. Parkinson, D.: Rapid serial simultaneous biplane stereoscopic angiography; an aid in the surgical management of cerebral arteriovenous malformations. Clin. Neurosurg. *16*, 179—184 (1969).

141. Parkinson, D.: Carotid Cavernous fistula: direct repair with preservation of the carotid artery. Technical note. J. Neurosurg. *38*, 99—106 (1973).

142. Parkinson, D., Legal, D., Holloway, A. F., *et al.*: A new combined neurosurgical headholder and cassette changer for intraoperative serial angiography. Technical note. J. Neurosurg. *48*, 1038—1041 (1978).

143. Peerless, S. J., Ferguson, G. G., Drake, C. G.: Extracranial-intracranial (EC/IC) bypass in the treatment of giant intracranial aneurysms. Neurosurg. Rev. *5*, 77—81 (1982).

144. Peronneau, P., Hinglais, J., Pellet, M., *et al.*: Vélocimètre sanguin par effet Doppler à émission ultrasonore pulsée. Onde électrique *50*, 369—384 (1970).

145. Pickard, J. D., Matheson, M., Patterson, J., *et al.*: Prediction of late ischemic complications after cerebral aneurysms surgery by the intraoperative measurement of cerebral blood flow. J. Neurosurg. *53*, 305—308 (1980).

146. Ploncard, P.: Some thoughts on extra-intracranial arterial bypass techniques. Acta Neurochir. (Wien) *50*, 229—236 (1979).

147. Pourcelot, L.: Applications cliniques de l'examen Doppler transcutané. Les colloques de l'Institut National de la Santé et de la Recherche Médicale. INSERM *34*, 213 (1974).

148. Reid, J. M.: Sound and ultrasound. In: Spencer, M. P., Reid, J. M. (eds.): Cerebrovascular Evaluation with Doppler Ultrasound, pp. 23—40. The Hague – Boston – London: Martinus Nijhoff, 1981.

149. Reneman, R. S.: Audio spectral analysis. In: Spencer, M. P., Reid, J. M. (eds.): Cerebrovascular Evaluation with Doppler Ultrasound, pp. 133—141. The Hague – Boston – London: Martinus Nijhoff, 1981.

150. Reneman, R. S., Hoeks, P. G.: Doppler Ultrasound in the Diagnosis of Cerebrovascular Disease. Chichester – New York – Brisbane – Toronto – Singapore: J. Wiley & Sons, 1982.

151. Reneman, R. S., Spencer, M. P.: Difficulties in processing of an analogue Doppler flow signal; with special reference to zero-crossing meters and quantification. In: Reneman, R. S. (ed.): Cardiovascular Applications of Ultrasound, pp. 32—42. Amsterdam – London: North-Holland Publishing Company, 1974.

152. Reneman, R. S., Spencer, M. P.: Local Doppler audio spectra in nor-

mal and stenosed carotid arteries in man. Ultrasound Med. Biol. *5*, 1—11 (1979).

153. von Reutern, G.-M., Büdingen, H. J., Hennerici, M., *et al.*: Diagnose und Differenzierung von Stenosen und Verschlüssen der Arteria carotis mit der Dopplersonographie. Arch. Psychiat. Nervenkr. *22*, 191—207 (1976).

154. von Reutern, G.-M., Voigt, K., Ortega-Suhrkamp, E., *et al.*: Dopplersonographische Befunde bei intrakraniellen vaskulären Störungen; Differentialdiagnose zu Obliterationen der extracraniellen Hirnarterien. Arch. Psychiat. Nervenkr. *223*, 1891—1896 (1977).

155. von Reutern, G.-M., Büdingen, H. J., Ortega-Suhrkamp, E., *et al.*: Differenzierungsmöglichkeiten der extrakraniellen Hirngefäße mit der Ultraschall-Doppler-Sonographie. In: Kriessmann, A., Bollinger, A. (eds.): Ultraschall-Doppler-Diagnostik in der Angiologie, pp. 105—113. Stuttgart – New York: G. Thieme, 1978.

156. von Reutern, G.-M., Pourcelot, L.: Cardiac cycle dependent alternating flow in vertebral arteries with subclavian artery stenoses. Stroke *9*, 229—236 (1978).

157. Robertson, J. H., Robertson, J. T.: The relationship between suture number and quality of anastomoses in microvascular procedures. Surg. Neurol. *10*, 241—245 (1978).

158. Rosenbaum, T. J., Sundt, T. M., Jr.: Neurovascular microsurgery, a model for laboratory investigation and the development of technical skills. Mayo Clin. Proc. *51*, 301—306 (1976).

159. Rosenbaum, T. J., Sundt, T. M., Jr.: Thrombus formation and endothelial alterations in microarterial anastomoses. J. Neurosurg. *47*, 430—441 (1977).

160. Roski, R. A., Spetzler, R. F., Nulsen, F. E.: Late complications of carotid ligation in the treatment of intracranial aneurysms. J. Neurosurg. *54*, 583—587 (1981).

161. Rushmer, R. F., Baker, D. W., Stegall, H. F.: Transcutaneous Doppler flow detection as a non-destructive technique. J. Appl. Physiol. *21*, 554 (1966).

162. Samson, D. S., Boone, S.: Extracranial-intracranial (EC-IC) arterial bypass: past performance and current concepts. Neurosurgery *3*, 79—86 (1978).

163. Santamore, W. P., Bove, A. A., Carey, R. A.: Hemodynamics of a stenosis in a complaint artery. Cardiology *69*, 1—10 (1982).

164. Satomura, S.: Ultrasonic Doppler method for the inspection of cardiac function. J. Acoust. Soc. Amer. *29*, 1181 (1957).

165. Satomura, S.: Study of the flow patterns in peripheral arteries by ultrasonics. J. Acoust. Soc. Jpn. *15*, 151—158 (1959).

166. Satomura, S., Kaneko, Z.: Ultrasonic blood rheograph. In: Proceedings of the 3rd International Conference of Medical Electronics. IEE, London, 1960, p. 254—258.

167. Schwartz, J. S., Carlyle, P. F., Cohn, J. N.: Effect of coronary arterial pressure on coronary artery stenosis. Circulation *61*, 70—76 (1980).

168. Shapiro, H. M., Stromberg, D. D., Lee, D. R., et al.: Dynamic pressures in the pial arterial microcirculation. Am. J. Physiol. 221, 279—283 (1971).
169. Shipley, R. E., Gregg, D. E.: The effect of external constriction of a blood vessel on blood flow. Am. J. Physiol. 141, 289—296 (1944).
170. Spencer, M. P., Reid, J. M.: Quantification of carotid stenosis with continuous-wave (C-W) Doppler ultrasound. Stroke 10, 326—330 (1979).
171. Spencer, M. P.: Hemodynamics of carotid artery stenosis. In: Spencer, M. P., Reid, J. M. (eds.): Cerebrovascular Evaluation with Doppler Ultrasound, pp. 114—131. The Hague - Boston - London: Martinus Nijhoff, 1981.
172. Spencer, M. P., Reid, J. M. (eds.): Cerebrovascular Evaluation with Doppler Ultrasound. The Hague - Boston - London: Martinus Nijhoff, 1981.
173. Spetzler, R. F., Chater, N.: Microvascular bypass surgery. Part 2: Physiological studies. J. Neurosurg. 45, 508—513 (1976).
174. Spetzler, R. F., Schuster, H., Roski, R. A.: Elective extracranial-intracranial arterial bypass in the treatment of inoperable giant aneurysms of the internal carotid artery. J. Neurosurg. 53, 22—27 (1980).
175. Spillner, G., Gonzales, J., von Reutern, G.-M.: The value of Doppler examination during and after surgery of the extracranial cerebral arteries. 9th International Salzburg Conference on Cerebral Vascular Disease, Salzburg, 1978.
176. Stegall, H. F., Rushmer, R. F., Baker, D. W.: A transcutaneous ultrasonic blood velocity meter. J. Appl. Physiol. 21, 707 (1966).
177. Stehbens, W. E.: Discussion on vascular flow and turbulence. Neurology (Minneap.) 11, 66—67 (1961).
178. Steiger, H. J.: Carotid Doppler hemodynamics in posttraumatic intracranial hypertension. Surg. Neurol. 16, 459—461 (1981).
179. Stephens, H. W., Jr.: Electromagnetic blood flowmetry in microvascular anastomosis. In: Fein, J. M., Reichman, O. H. (eds.): Microvascular Anastomoses for Cerebral Ischemia, pp. 181—194. Berlin - Heidelberg - New York: Springer, 1978.
180. Stephens, H. W.: Measurement of intracranial arterial pressure in patients undergoing extracranial to intracranial microsurgical anastomosis for cerebrovascular ischemia. In: Peerless, S. J., McCormick, C. W. (eds.): Microsurgery for Cerebral Ischemia, pp. 252—256. Berlin - Heidelberg - New York: Springer, 1980.
181. Strandness, D. E., Jr., McCutcheon, E. P., Rushmer, R. F.: Application of a transcutaneous Doppler flowmeter in evaluation of occlusive arterial disease. Surg. Gynec. Obstet. 22, 1039 (1966).
182. Strandness, D. E., Jr., Sumner, D. S.: Clinical applications of continous wave and pulsed Doppler velocity detectors. INSERM 34, 147—190 (1974).
183. Stromberg, P. D., Fox, J. R.: Pressure in the pial arterial microcircu-

lation of the cat during changes in systemic arterial blood pressure. Circ. Res. *31,* 229—239 (1972).

184. Sundt, T. M., Sharbrough, F. W., Anderson, R. E., *et al.*: Cerebral blood flow measurements and electroencephalograms during carotid endarterectomy. J. Neurosurg. *41,* 310—320 (1974).

185. Sundt, T. M., Sandok, B. A., Whisnant, J. P.: Carotid endarterectomy: Complications and preoperative assessment of risk. Mayo Clin. Proc. *50,* 301—306 (1975).

186. Sundt, T. M., Kobayashi, S., Fode, N. C., *et al.*: Results and complications of surgical mangement of 809 intracranial aneurysms in 722 cases. J. Neurosurg. *56,* 753—765 (1982).

187. Thal, T.-U.: Evaluation of patency during and after extracranial-intracranial bypass operations using Doppler sonography. In: Dietz, H., Metzel, E., Langmaid, C. (eds.): Neurological Surgery, Supplement to Neurochirurgia, p. 384. Stuttgart – New York: G. Thieme, 1981.

188. Thompson, J. R., Rouhe, S. A., Austin, G. M., *et al.*: Angiographic cerebral blood flow patterns in STA-MCA anastomosis candidates. In: Fein, J. M., Reichman, O. H. (eds.): Microvascular Anastomosis for Cerebral Ischemia, pp. 145—157. Berlin – Heidelberg – New York: Springer, 1978.

189. Tsitsopoulos, P., Malbouisson, M. B., Harrison, M. J. G.: End-to-side vascular anastomosis: a study of technical considerations in the rat. J. Neurosurg. *56,* 642—645 (1982).

190. Tulleken, C. A. F., Hoogland, P., Sloof, J.: A new technique for the end-to-end anastomosis between small arteries. In: Peerless, S. J., McCormick, C. W.: Microsurgery for Cerebral Ischemia, pp. 173—177. Berlin – Heidelberg – New York: Springer, 1980.

191. Wassmann, H., Fischdick, G., Holbach, K.-H.: Ultrasonic Doppler assessment of hemodynamics in extra-intracranial arterial bypass (EIAB) surgery. 5th International Symposion on Microvascular Anastomoses for Cerebral Ischemia (abstr.). Wien, 1980, p. 85.

192. Weir, B., Grace, M., Hansen, J., *et al.*: Time course of vasospasm in man. J. Neurosurg. *48,* 173—178 (1978).

193. Weir, B.: Value of immediate postoperative angiography following aneurysm surgery. J. Neurosurg. *54,* 396—398 (1981).

194. Weissenhofer, W., Schmidt, R., Schenck, W. G., Jr.: Technique of electromagnetic blood flow measurements: notes, regarding a potential source of error. Surgery *73,* 474—477 (1973).

195. Wells P. N. T.: The possibility of harmful biological effects in ultrasonic diagnosis. In: Reneman, R. S. (ed.): Cardiovascular Applications of Ultrasound, pp. 1—17. Amsterdam – London: North-Holland Publishing Company 1974.

196. Wells, P. N. T.: Physical principles of ultrasonic diagnosis. New York – London: Academic Press, 1969.

197. Wieslander, J. B., Aberg, M.: Blood flow in small arteries after

end-to-end and end-in-end anastomoses: an experimental quantitative comparison. J. Microsurg. *2*, 121—125 (1980).

198. Wieslander, J. B., Aberg, M.: Stenosis following end-in-end microarterial anastomosis: an angiographic comparison with the end-to-end technique. J. Microsurg. *3*, 151—155 (1982).

199. Wilkins, D. G., Cummins, B. H., Griffith, H. B., *et al.*: Repeated measurements of cerebral blood flow during intracranial surgery. Lancet *2*, 402—403 (1972).

200. Wille, S. O., Walloe, L.: Pulsatile pressure and flow in arterial stenoses simulated in an mathematical model. J. Biomed. Engng. *3*, 17—24 (1981).

201. Wollschlaeger, G., Wollschlaeger, P. B.: The Circle of Willis. In: Newton, T. H., Potts, D. G.: Radiology of the Skull and Brain; Vol. 2, Book 2, pp. 1171—1201. St. Louis: C. V. Mosby, 1974.

202. Woodhall, B., Odom, G. L., Bloor, B. M., *et al.*: Direct measurement of intravascular pressure in components of the circle of Willis. A contribution to the surgery of congenital cerebral aneurysms and vascular anomalies of the brain. Ann. Surg. *135*, 911—921 (1952).

203. Yashon, D., Magness, A. P., Vise, W. M.: Systemic hypotension in neurosurgery. J. Neurosurg. *43*, 579—589 (1975).

204. Yonekawa, Y., Yaşargil, M. G.: Extra-intracranial arterial anastomosis: clinical and technical aspects. Results. In: Krayenbuehl, H., *et al.* (eds.): Advances and Technical Standards in Neurosurgery, Vol. 3, pp. 47—78. Wien – New York: Springer, 1976.

205. Yongchareon, W., Young, D. F.: Initiation of turbulence in models of arterial stenoses. J. Biomechanics *12*, 185—196 (1979).

Subject Index

W. Seeger, University of Freiburg i. Br.

Microsurgery of the Cranial Base

1983. 200 figures. Approx. 400 pages.
Format: 24,2 cm × 31,2 cm.
ISBN 3-211-81769-7

"Microsurgery of the Cranial Base" is a continuation of the critically acclaimed "Microsurgery of the Brain". In this new book you will find the same clear format and the same meticulous presentation of technical principles in conjunction with detailed anatomical overviews. You will also find outstanding illustrations by the author that help bring you closer to a three-dimensional orientation.

The main focus of this volume is upon tumors and vascular processes in the areas of basal dura and dura duplicatures, particularly on their relations to cranial nerves and basal vessels. Oronasal hypophysis operations − with special anatomical aspects and variants − as well as processes in the Sinus cavernosus area are emphasized.

The first half of the book will be of particular interest to otorhinolaryngologists and ophthalmologists because it focuses on the operative approaches and processes in the Sinus and orbita transition area. Operations in the area of A. carotis int. (i.e. ophthalmic aneurysms) are also included since they often necessitate simultaneous bypass-operations. Here, Dr. Seeger also introduces the use of preoperative Doppler-sonographic checks.

Possible problems involving the Os ethmoides and Sinus frontalis are demonstrated on a problematic frontobasal fracture and Olfactorius meningioma. Descriptions of decompression of nerves and vessels in the posterior fossa are included.

The book concludes with an examination of the technical and anatomical problems caused by tumors displacing the Sinus sigmoideus and Sulcus sigmoideus.

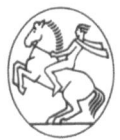

Springer-Verlag Wien New York

W. Seeger

Microsurgery of the Spinal Cord and Surrounding Structures

Anatomical and Technical Principles

1982. 201 figures. VII, 410 pages.
Format: 24,2 cm × 31,2 cm.
ISBN 3-211-81648-8

Distribution rights for Japan: Nankodo Co. Ltd., Tokyo

This book is primarily concerned with operative interventions of extra and intradural tumors, angiomas, and malformations of the spinal canal (and some typical lesions occurring there). Since Dr. Seeger believes that a thorough familiarity with topographical anatomy is a prerequisite to successful microsurgery, precise anatomical models of each procedure are provided. These help to elucidate the principles of the operation as well as depict neighboring structures generally not visible from the surgeon's perspective, but which nevertheless can play an important role in a particular maneuver.

Microsurgery of the Brain

Anatomical and Technical Principles

1980. 351 figures. XI, IV, 727 pages.
Format: 24,2 cm × 31,2 cm.
In two volumes, not sold separately.
ISBN 3-211-81573-2

Distribution rights for Japan: Nankodo Co. Ltd., Tokyo

Atlas of Topographical Anatomy of the Brain and Surrounding Structures

for Neurosurgeons, Neuroradiologists, and Neuropathologists

1978. 258 figures. IX, 544 pages.
Format: 24,2 cm × 31,2 cm.
ISBN 3-211-81447-7

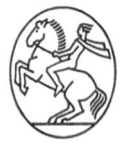

**Springer-Verlag
Wien New York**

Distribution rights for Japan: Nankodo Co. Ltd., Tokyo
Distribution rights for Socialist Countries: J. A. Barth, Leipzig